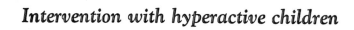
Intervention with hyperactive children

Principles and techniques of intervention with hyperactive children

Edited by

MARVIN J. FINE, Ph. D.

School of Education
University of Kansas
Lawrence, Kansas

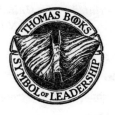

CHARLES C THOMAS · PUBLISHER
Springfield · Illinois · U.S.A.

Published and Distributed Throughout the World by
CHARLES C THOMAS • PUBLISHER
BANNERSTONE HOUSE
301-327 East Lawrence Avenue, Springfield, Illinois, U.S.A.

© *1977, by* CHARLES C THOMAS • PUBLISHER
ISBN 0-398-03570-9
Library of Congress Catalog Card Number 76-8230

Printed in the United States of America
N-1

Library of Congress Cataloging in Publication Data

Main entry under title:

Principles and techniques of intervention wth hyperactive children.

  Bibliography: p.
  Includes index.
  1. Hyperactive children. 2. Psychotherapy. I. Fine, Marvin J. II. Title:
Intervention with hyperactive children.
RJ506.H9P74   618.9'28'58   76-8230
ISBN 0-398-03570-9

Contributors

Norma J. Dyck, Ph.D.
Project Coordinator, Comprehensive Personnel Planning for Handicapped in Kansas
Lawrence, Kansas

Marvin J. Fine, Ph.D.
Professor, Department of Educational Psychology and Research
University of Kansas
Lawrence, Kansas

Mary Mira, Ph.D.
Associate Professor, Department of Psychology
University of Kansas Medical Center
Kansas City, Kansas

John P. Poggio, Ph.D.
Associate Professor, Department of Educational Psychology and Research
University of Kansas
Lawrence, Kansas

Carol Ann Reece, M.D.
Gardner Medical Center
Gardner, Kansas

Herbert J. Rieth, Ed.D.
Research Associate, Bureau of Child Research

University of Kansas
Lawrence, Kansas

Neil J. Salkind, Ph.D.
Assistant Professor, Department of Educational Psychology and Research
University of Kansas
Lawrence, Kansas

Richard L. Simpson, Ed.D.
Assistant Professor, Department of Special Education
University of Kansas Medical Center
Kansas City, Kansas

Alice Vlietstra, Ph.D.
Assistant Professor, Department of Psychology
University of Missouri at St. Louis

Clifton W. Wolf, Ph.D.
Clinical Psychologist
Kansas City, Missouri

John C. Wright, Ph.D.
Professor, Department of Human Development
Department of Psychology
University of Kansas
Lawrence, Kansas

DEDICATED
to the memory of my father,
Samuel Fine.

Preface

T HIS COLLECTION of writings on the hyperactive child attempts to offer a concise and critical presentation of concepts and research findings and, most importantly, of different viewpoints on intervention. There is far from concensus on many facets of hyperactivity, and this book will identify and elucidate some of the controversies. Many of the voices being expressed on the topic resound with surety; the thinking on hyperactivity has periodically become simplistic in the search for a *cause* and a *cure*. For some people the label of *brain damage* has become a unitary cause and explanation catch-all term. Some others identify with the singular notions of temperament, diet or history of faulty reinforcement as explanations of the cause and developmental progress of hyperactivity. The potentialities for causes and for influencers of subsequent development are great, with many factors likely interacting to produce an effect. If final answers were indeed available, then hyperactivity would cease to exist as a major problem for children, parents and teachers.

The several contributors represent different disciplines and theoretical orientations but are all concerned with the welfare of the hyperactive child. They recognize the cruciality of the school experience for this child, and they have been willing to present their viewpoints on his behalf and to challenge existing beliefs and practices when necessary.

The first chapter will review basic information, beliefs and procedures, setting the stage for the subsequent chapters. Specifically, the introductory chapter will present definitial and conceptual viewpoints and problems, incidence figures, data on the development course of hyperactivity, a review of causal factors and of intervention-treatment approaches.

The chapter on medical management attempts to put in a realistic perspective what medical treatment has to offer and how physicians and educators can cooperate. The views presented in this chapter are backed by the extensive involvement of Dr. Mira, a psychologist, and Dr. Reece, a pediatrician, in the treatment of hyperactive children. Both hold appointments at the University of Kansas Medical Center.

Dr. Herbert Rieth's chapter on behavioral management reviews and illustrates specific applications of behavior modification with hyperactive children. This chapter is enriched by the sharing of studies completed by classroom teachers. A former teacher and school psychologist who is currently involved in school psychological consultation and behavioral research, Dr. Rieth brings much first-hand experience with hyperactive children to his chapter.

The fourth chapter on educational management by Dr. Norma Dyck will attend directly to the curricular and classroom organizational patterns. Her chapter examines educational management from differing positions including behavioral engineering and neuroeducationally-based approaches. The writings of Frank Hewitt and William Cruickshank are prominent in the chapter. Her own background as a classroom teacher, learning disabilities consultant and director of a project focussing on offering support to teachers, has sensitized Dr. Dyck to the classroom problem presented by hyperactive children.

Dr. Clifton Wolf is a clinical psychologist who formerly taught in the public schools and directed a reading clinic. He is actively involved in transactional analysis and is a Provisional Teaching Member of the International Transactional Analysis Association. Dr. Wolf's chapter introduces the reader to basic T.A. theory and methods, and illustrates the applications to both understanding the hyperactive child and to helping the child manage his own behavior.

A more complete understanding of hyperactivity in children requires knowledge of the normal variances in child development. Drs. John Wright and Alice Vlietstra present their research on cognitive tempo in children, focussing on the dimensions of impulsivity and reflectivity. This chapter becomes important background for those concerned with hyperactivity who wish to add a child development dimension to their clinical or educational orientation.

The definition and measurement of a variable would logically seem necessary for the systematic study of that variable. As the chapter by Drs. Salkind and Poggio reveals, definition and measurement have been crucial problem areas with the study of hyperactivity. Their chapter serves as a rich source of ideas and suggestions in this area.

The annotated bibliography prepared by Dr. Richard Simpson offers the reader a current extensive overview of research and writings on hyperactivity. This chapter concisely summarizes many of the studies mentioned in the respective chapters and introduces the reader to additional studies and articles.

MARVIN J. FINE, *Editor*
University of Kansas
Lawrence, Kansas

Contents

Intervention with hyperactive children

1

Hyperactivity: where are we?

Marvin J. Fine

HYPERACTIVITY is one of the most frequently cited symptoms of children referred by parents or teachers for professional help. As a symptom it has been commonly associated with categories of emotional disturbance, learning disabilities and neurological impairment. It has even found its way into legitimization as a syndrome, *hyperkinetic impulse disorder,* while other authorities have argued the existence of several discernible kinds of hyperactivity.

Paradoxically, despite the seeming concensus on associating the symptom with pathological conditions, there remains substantial divergence of opinion regarding the etiology, epidemiology, developmental course and treatment procedures of hyperactivity. Viewed as either symptom or syndrome, it has provoked a democratic outpouring of interest from medicine, pharmacology, education and psychology. Irate parent and civil rights groups should also be included in the potpourri of interested parties in relation to charges of drugging hyperactive children into more submissive states.

3

Numerous questions are raised when a child seems to be hyperactive:

Is the child really hyperactive or just a child with a lot of energy?
Should he be referred for medical study?
Will drugs slow him down physically but still permit him to learn?
Can we use behavior modification to reduce his hyperactivity?
Will putting him in a cubicle help him to attend and learn?
Are we inadvertently *programming* the child to be hyperactive?
Is the child constitutionally impulsive, and should we permit the child to function *his way?*
If we can tolerate the child now, will he outgrow the *condition* by puberty?

School personnel have been particularly sensitized to hyperactive children because of the difficulties of managing them in a classroom setting. The normal dilemma of diagnosis and management becomes accentuated given the interaction of the child with the variables inherent in any classroom. For example, teaching style, curricular organization, teacher values and peer factors all interact with the child's adjustment and learning potential.

The concern of educators with extremely physically active children is hardly a recent phenomenon. In 1803, Joseph Lancaster, a London schoolmaster, presented his innovations for disciplining "wrongdoers" (Emblen, 1969). One of his proposals was the "log." This involved balancing a four to six-pound log on the child's shoulders while looping a cord over the child's head. If the child figited or squirmed, the log would slip off the shoulders, thereby, putting it mildly, causing the neck to smart. Lancaster also described the use of "the schackle," a wood and rope device that would hobble a child, reducing his ability to move about quickly. If this did not succeed in slowing down and controlling the child's movements, Lancaster offered several other suggestions, including actually tying the child's legs together.

It would be falsely reassuring to believe that such procedures are totally a thing of the past. A recent excellent and comprehensive review of corporal punishment (Mauer, 1974) made it dramatically evident that inappropriate, sadistic and peculiar methods are still being used actively in the schools to manage the behavior of children. This mention of the continued existence of extreme measures to control children was not meant as an indictment of teachers but rather to highlight the degree of frustration and impotence that many teachers feel when attempting to cope with an excessively physically active child. The writer knows of kindergarten teachers who have tied children to their seats and of a teacher who put an older boy on a leash, one end to the desk and one to the child's foot; both of those moves were desperate attempts by the teachers to control the physical activity of the child.

The demands made on teachers are surely excessive when viewed by any reasonable standard. Teachers are expected to prepare lesson plans not only for a total class but for individual and subgroupings of children within the classroom based on those children's specific educational and personal needs. Teachers are expected to cope with the personal and social adjustment needs of children, helping isolates to socialize, converting the bullies into leaders, *me-first* children into sharers and day dreamers into motivated learners. Is it any wonder that children who are chronically figiting, distracted, impulsive and emotionally labile take on a special negative significance to many teachers?

"Hyperactive children by reason of their concommitant learning and management problems constitute one of the most perplexing issues to teachers and administrators and indeed to emotionally normal children within the school" (Cruickshank, 1967 p. 48). The teacher's frustration is often further amplified by either the absence of any outside assistance, such as a concerned physician or school psychologist, or by the seemingly inappropriate recommendations of experts who appear unaware of the realities of the classroom. It is infuriating to have persons the teacher turns to for help either parrot back in *jargoneez* exactly what the teacher initially reported on the child, or to have the person present a complex and seemingly inapplicable set of directives.

One psychiatrist used to ask the teacher what had worked, even a little. Once this information had been obtained on some last ditch, marginally successful ploy, he would glibly advise the teacher, "Well, that sounds good; keep trying it." Needless to say, he was not the teacher's favorite referral resource.

WHAT IS A HYPERACTIVE CHILD?

One team of researchers acknowledged that there was much confusion and disagreement, vagueness and subjectivity regarding the term *hyperactivity,* and they concluded, "It is our impression that hyperactivity describes those aspects of a person's behavior which annoy the observer" (Buddenhagen and Sickler, 1969 p. 580). Probably, the most defensible definition of a hyperactive child would have to be simply "a child that some authority labels as being hyperactive."

Because such disciplines as medicine, psychology and education have all been concerned with this child, the definitions that have appeared in the literature have tended to reflect the viewpoints of the disciplines as well as different theoretical orientations such as neurological, psychological and behavioral. In a recent article, Delong (1972) commented that there are at least thirty-seven different labels on terms used, with the terms hyperactivity, hyperkinesis, hyperkinetic impulse disorder, and minimal brain dysfunction (MBD) being the most common. Many such terms are used interchangeably, and even when some differentiation is attempted, there is much overlap.

The salient behavioral characteristics of hyperactivity were presented by one writer as:

1. short attention span;
2. restlessness and overactivity (motor driveness) ;
3. poor judgment;
4. low frustration tolerance and irritability;
5. poor perceptual and conceptual abilities;
   (reflected in serious academic deficiencies) ;
6. defective memory;
7. poor muscular coordination.

(Burks, 1960 p. 18)

From a study wherein mothers were interviewed regarding their child's behavior, Stewart (1970) reported the most prominent symptoms being "overactive, doesn't finish projects, figits, can't sit still at meals, doesn't stay with games, talks too much, doesn't follow directions" and "clumsy." These symptoms ranged from 62 percent of the children on "clumsy" and "doesn't follow directions," up to 84 percent on "figits" and "doesn't finish projects," and 100 percent on "overactive."

Another definition was proposed by Chess (1960) who viewed the hyperactive child as "one who carries out activities at a higher rate of speed than the average child, or is constantly in motion, or both" (Chess, 1960 p. 2379). The consideration of higher-than-average activity level has been utilized by many other writers. One of the most prolific contributors to the literature on hyperactivity has defined developmental hyperactivity as:

> . . . a level of daily motor activity which is clearly greater (ideally by more than two standard deviations from the mean) than that occurring in children of similar sex, mental age, socioeconomic and cultural background and which is not accompanied by clear evidence of major central nervous system disorder or childhood psychosis and which has been present consistently since the earliest years of life.
>
> (Werry, 1968 p. 583)

Werry was accepting of an organically-based hyperactivity, but felt it important to distinguish a syndrome of hyperactivity that appeared developmental in nature and not connected to a condition of brain damage.

A survey completed among teachers, psychologists, psychiatrists, social workers and pediatricians did reveal good agreement on the behavioral characteristics of hyperactivity:

> Seventy-five percent or more of all groups felt the following six behaviors to be primary: figits and restless, inattentive, hard to manage, can't sit still, easily distracted, and low frustration. Medical professionals were concerned also with irritability, undisciplined, clumsy, poor sleeper, seems slow and awkward.
>
> (Schrager, Lindy, Harrison,
> McDermott and Killins, 1966 p. 636)

In reviewing the plethora of available definitions, Simpson and Nelson (1974) identified two primary aspects of symptom patterns. The first pattern involved references to activity level. From the definitions that were just reviewed this pattern becomes evident with the focus on "higher than average" physical activity. The second pattern was seen as involving the situational or social appropriateness of the child's motor behavior. In some situations or environments a great deal of motor behavior is more acceptable, tolerated or even encouraged. In other settings or on other occasions, appropriateness requires a lower level of motor behavior.

The answer to the question "What is a hyperactive child?" should include a theoretical concept of hyperactivity, a behavioral description of the pattern or patterns of hyperactivity, and, finally, systematic procedures for assessing the hyperactivity. The literature reviewed thus far would seem to indicate that the greatest agreement among professionals is on the behavioral characteristics of hyperactivity. There is greater diversity of opinion on the theoretical concept of hyperactivity and on assessment procedures. The chapter by Salkind and Poggio entitled "The Measurement of Hyperactivity: Trends and Issues" will examine more closely the problems involved in conceptualizing and measuring hyperactivity. The interested reader is also referred to the annotated bibliography prepared by Richard Simpson for additional literature on the measurement of hyperactivity.

HOW FREQUENT IS HYPERACTIVITY?

Obviously, any survey on the frequency of a phenomenon should start with a common definition. Since there is not a common definition despite general agreement on primary symptoms, we can expect to hear differing incidence figures on hyperactivity. Nonetheless, the figures that are reported all substantiate the picture of a large number of children experiencing the various symptoms of hyperactivity. Eisenberg (1973), for example, reported that there are between 500,000 and 1.5 million hyperkinetic children of elementary school age in the United States.

A 1971 conference on stimulant medications sponsored by the Department of Health, Education and Welfare (reported in the *Journal of Learning Disabilities,* 1971, volume 4, p. 523) offered a conservative estimate of 3 percent of all elementary school children as experiencing moderate and severe hyperkinetic disorders. Other figures of 4 to 8 percent (Stewart, Pitts, Craig, and Dieruf, 1966) and 10 percent (Huessy, 1967) have also been presented.

When the starting point for incidence figures is an atypical population, the incidence figures soar. Rogers, Lilienfeld and Pasamanick (1955) reported that approximately 40 percent of children referred to mental health clinics exhibit hyperkinetic behavior. In a study examining behavior patterns of learning disability children (Paraskevopoulos and McCarthy, 1970), hyperactivity was a part of the most frequently occurring pattern of behavior. Furthermore, teachers and mothers had a high degree of agreement in their ratings of the children's behavior. The incidence figures rise among the mentally retarded population as testified to by Horenstein's (1957) description of hyperactivity as the most serious management problem in institutions for retarded children. A recent study (Keogh, Tchir, and Windeguth-Behn, 1974) identified hyperactivity as the most frequently mentioned descriptor by teachers describing characteristics of educationally handicapped children.

The incidence of hyperactivity among identified brain damaged children is perhaps the most difficult statistic to obtain with any accuracy, since for many clinicians the symptom of hyperactivity is used as one of the indicators of brain damage. Hyperkinetic behavior in children came under scrutiny following the 1918 epidemic of encephalitis in the United States. Many of the children who had contracted encephalitis later showed personality and behavior changes, including becoming hyperactive. This observation, along with the recognition that other children with identifiable brain damage also experienced hyperactivity, precipitated the association of hyperactivity with brain damage. This connection however is one of the areas of strong disagreement among clinicians and researchers as will be discussed later.

Chess (1960) reported 15 percent of hyperactive children having minimal cerebral dysfunction while McIntosh and Dunn (1973) concluded from their review of the relevant literature that noticeable hyperactivity occurred in only about 20 percent of school children who had been classified as brain injured. It is interesting to note how the term *only* is often used in describing the incidence of hyperactive, brain damaged children. This is in deference to those whose orientation to hyperactivity would argue a higher relationship.

The incidence figures seem to vary as a function of the definition of hyperactivity, how it was measured and the population sampled. For supposedly normal populations, the estimates seem to range from 3 to 10 percent. For already identified *problem* populations such as emotionally disturbed, mentally retarded, learning disabled and brain damaged, the most frequently cited figures run from 10 to 20 percent. As with many *problem* conditions, boys again markedly predominate over girls.

This ratio ranges from a low of 2-5 boys to every girl, through a more common proportion of four to six boys to every girl, up to a high figure of nine boys to every girl. These findings mirror the preponderance of boys seen with such disorders as autism, reading disability, and delayed speech development.

(Stewart and Olds, 1973 p. 19)

WHAT IS THE DEVELOPMENTAL COURSE OF HYPERACTIVITY?

Some years ago the writer was present when a noted medical expert, tongue-in-cheek, advised school psychologists to begin working with hyperactive children as they were reaching puberty (the children, not the psychologists). His point was that hyperactivity will subside as a natural function of the maturing child and the psychologist would then appear skilled, knowledgeable and a real expert. Several researchers and clinicians (Werry, 1968; Laufer, 1972; Solomons, 1965; and Minde, Lewin, Weiss, Lavigueur, Douglas, and Sykes, 1971) have either reported data or opinion on the longevity of hyperactivity and basically concur with its diminishment concurrent with pubescence. Laufer (1972) advised physicians, "It can be stated with confidence that the hyperkinetic syndrome of behavior will be outgrown—treated or untreated—when the child is between 12 and 18 years of age. As yet there is no way of predicting for a given individual when this favorable outcome will occur." (Laufer, 1972 p. 230). Laufer cautioned however that the certitude of the prediction applied only to the symptoms of hyperkinesis and not necessarily to the emotional or learning problem aspects of the condition.

Children whose classroom adjustment has been negatively affected because of their hyperkinesis logically would have difficulties in achievement, peer relationships and self-concept. Some professionals have preferred to view the so-called hyperactive child as really a child with a lot of energy who conceivably could grow up as an enthusiastic, active person rather than someone with problems. There unquestionably are children with higher-than-average energy levels who nonetheless are able to concentrate, are not irritable or emotionally labile, do not have fine motor problems and in fact are adjusting quite adequately. But the child viewed as hyperactive usually is in conflict with his environment, be it parents, teachers or peers and may not just outgrow his problems.

A recent study (Minde et al., 1971) revealed some pessimistic follow-up information on hyperactive children. This well-designed study included thirty-seven children with an average age of twelve years who four to six years earlier had been identified as hyperactive. These students were paired with a child of the same sex in his classroom and the two groups, hyperactives and normals, then compared across several variables. The hyperactive children repeated more grades than the normal children and also scored significantly lower in all subjects except art, handwork and physical activity. The mean IQ of the hyperactive children was also significantly lower than that of the control group, but still fell within the average range of intelligence. The researchers recognized that there were problems with the IQ score; for example, did the hyperactive behavior interfere with test performance? But even when twenty-three of the hyperactive children were matched on IQ with control children, the achievement level of hyperactives was still significantly lower. The hyperactive children were also rated by their teachers as presenting significantly more behavior problems than control children. Other studies (Laufer, 1962; Loney, 1974; and Menkes, Rowe and Menkes, 1967) have supported the picture of continued adjustment and learning problems with age and after the more prominent symptoms of hyperactivity subside.

In summary, while the physical manifestations of hyperactivity may reduce with adolescence, the hyperactive child often has a history of lower academic achievement and social problems that still affect his overall adjustment, ". . . hyperactivity . . . is a condition which profoundly affects the personal and academic life of the individual child and requires long term psychological, academic, and remedial assistance." (Minde, et al., 1971 p. 221).

The follow-up data being reported by Minde was normative in the sense that it depicted how the children developed in the absence of major attempts to directly help them, the parents or the educational setting. If such data were favorable, then the hyperactive child would be in fine shape, and this book would be unnecessary. Hopefully, through the continued efforts of professionals and with the selective application of preventive and remedial strategies, the developmental course of specific hyperactive children will be more favorable.

IS THERE A RELATIONSHIP BETWEEN HYPERACTIVITY AND LEARNING PROBLEMS?

There seems to be general agreement that hyperactive children as a group do experience school learning difficulties. While admittedly there may be periodic confusion between *how the child performs* and *what the child knows,* there is an accumulation of evidence supporting the existence of learning problems. Following a review of the school behaviors of hyperactive children, Douglas (1972 p. 261) reported there was ". . . a high incidence of failed grades among the hyperactives. By the time they were 12 years of age, 70 percent of them had failed one year, and 20 percent had failed two years. The hyperactive children also had significantly lower grades than the controls on almost all academic subjects."

There is a lack of concensus however on what is the exact nature of the learning difficulties. For example, Freibergs and Douglas (1969) reported that hyperactive children performed as well as a normal sample on concept-learning tasks under the condition of a continuous reinforcement schedule. Under the condition of partial reinforcement the hyperactive children's quality of performance decreased. These authors speculated that the performance difficulties that hyperactive children experience in school situations might be more a function of attentional and motivational variables than of specific cognitive impairments. The suggestion that follows these findings is to structure the school learning experience with continuous reinforcement to maintain the child attending to task. An excellent paper by Alabiso (1972) also focussed on the importance of increasing attention in hyperactive children through systematic reinforcement.

A somewhat different view of how hyperactivity interferes with school learning was discussed by Cruickshank (1967) who described two interrelated aspects of hyperactivity, those of a sensory and of a motoric nature. The child with a sensory hyperactivity will experience difficulty attending to a single stimulus or a group of stimuli for a needed length of time. He may also have difficulty in differentiating foreground from background and in conceptualizing the relationship among parts of a task and the total task. The child may also have difficulty with spatial orientation, shifting from line to line or skipping problems. Additionally, the child may have a tendency to perseverate as shown, for example, by his inability to shift from addition to subtraction in a series of problems. These characteristics denote impaired cognitive functioning beyond the notion postulated by others of an attention deficit.

The second main aspect of hyperactivity that Cruickshank (1967 p. 57) presented, motor disinhibition, was described as ". . . the inability of the child to refrain from reacting to a stimulus which produces a motor response. Anything which can be pulled, turned, pushed, twisted, bent, torn, wiggled, scratched, or otherwise manipulated motorically will be so handled." Either sensory or motor hyperactivity, but especially the two in combination, is likely to substantially interfere with school learning.

Keogh (1971), in her review of the literature on hyperactivity and learning disorders, identified three main hypotheses. Hypothesis 1 was that neurological impairment explained the learning problems found in hyperactive children. She viewed the controversial and confusing drug research with hyperactive children as indirectly supporting this hypothesis—that is, if medication leads to improvement in learning, then this infers that the initial problem was organic in nature. However, as Keogh herself points out, "It appears likely that medication may affect change in level of motor activity and in attention, but that the direct effect of medication on learning is unclear. Change in behavior in a more socially compatible direction, however, may be an extremely significant factor in learning success. In this sense medication may indirectly facilitate improvement in learning." (Keogh, 1971 p. 103)." She concluded that while the neurological hypothesis was reasonable as a possible explanation for the behavior of hyperactive children, it was unacceptable as a basic explanation for learning problems these children experience.

The second hypothesis reviewed was concerned with information acquisition. This line of reasoning was that the motor activity the hyperactive child manifests interferes with attention to task, and necessarily then with the initial acquisition of information. The focus here as discussed earlier is on the capacity of the child to attend. The evidence of hyperactive children performing well on concept tasks under conditions of continuous reinforcement would support the plausibility of this hypothesis. The chapters by Herbert Rieth and Norma Dyck will address themselves in part to the question of "How do you obtain and maintain the child's attention?"

The third hypothesis Keogh considered was that the hyperactive child is a faulty decision maker. The emphasis was on the excessive speed with which the child made his decisions, often appearing impulsive when some reflection was necessary. The work of Kagan (1966) was cited to support this position. Other data was presented to illustrate that when these children slow down their response rate and spend more time in scanning the task, the level of performance increased. The chapter by John Wright and Alice Vlietstra will look more fully at the differences in children along the dimensions of impulsivity and reflectivity, how these cognitive patterns affect learning, and whether the patterns can and should be modified.

In summary, hyperactive children as a group do experience below-average school achievement, but the exact nature of the learning difficulties is not established. Just as the causes of hyperactivity appear to be diverse and multiple, so does it seem logical that the causes and manifestations of learning difficulties may vary considerably among hyperactive children.

WHAT CAUSES HYPERACTIVITY?

A review of the literature on causal factors highlights three main causal considerations—organic, developmental and psychological. However, even the staunchest proponent of a single *main cause* theory will acknowledge the importance of the child in interaction with his environment. But before looking at such interaction, let us first review each of the three basic positions.

Organically Caused Hyperactivity

As mentioned earlier, a relationship was noted between encephalitis and hyperactivity (Ebaugh, 1923 and Kahn and Cohen, 1934) that prompted a flow of research and hypothesizing regarding how to medically and educationally manage these children. Strauss and Lehtinen (1948) and Strauss and Kephart (1955) viewed hyperactivity as a product of minimal brain damage and produced a philosophy of educational programming that while achieving some popularity, remained basically controversial. Cruickshank has carried forward this etiological theme in his statements on hyperactivity (1967) but has acknowledged that existing diagnostic instrumentation may not be adequate to prove this relationship. His conviction, which is well shared by many others, is conveyed in his positing that when appropriate instrumentation is available, "We shall undoubtedly see that most if not all hyperactive children have a specific neurological basis to their behavior," (Cruickshank, 1967). Solomons, (1971 p. 472) another important contributor to the literature on hyperactivity made a similar observation in regard to the use of medication with these children, "The 'hyperkinetic impulse disorder' is a recognizable clinical entity and falls within the overall category of minimal cerebral dysfunction on an organic basis. Although we have not definitely proved this point, we have the impression that by classifying increased activity in this way, we can better select the medication of choice."

There has in fact been a developing body of evidence pointing to the organic basis of hyperactivity, but the evidence by virtue of its manner of being obtained and its lack of conclusiveness still leaves the relationship between hyperactivity and organic factors a debatable issue.

Typical of the kind of findings that often occur, is the medical evaluation data reported on one hundred children who were referred to a clinic with one of the presenting complaints being hyperactivity (Kenny, Clemmens, Hudson, Lentz, Cicci, and Nair, 1971). In over half of the group, neurological findings were normal. None of the children were unequivocably judged to be neurologically abnormal while *soft* neurological signs were found in forty-eight children. Of the seventy-eight children who were also given electroencephalograms, thirty-eight were normal. The authors also reported disconcertingly that a significant relationship was not found among the neurological examination, electroencephalographic findings and the final diagnosis. Further complicating these data was the fact that only thirty-five of the one hundred children were judged by a majority of the clinical team to actually be hyperactive.

A key difficulty with the organic etiology category is that it may encompass a variety of divergent etiological factors from major to minimal brain damage, specific to diffuse brain damage and biochemical factors influencing brain functioning. This in turn means that a group of children with established or strongly suspected brain damage will probably be quite heterogeneous in many respects. Conners (1973) reported data to support this notion. He was able to identify six group profiles from a sample of children purported to have minimal brain dysfunction. Each subgroup was established on the basis of the variables of general IQ, achievement, rote learning, attentiveness and impulse control.

Another problem as earlier mentioned is the apparent lack of adequate refinement in the diagnostic instrumentation needed to pinpoint organic factors. Additionally, some circularity of reasoning has persisted which has not added any light to the problem: (a) Hyperactivity can be caused by brain damage; (b) hyperactivity is one diagnostic indicator of brain damage; (c) the existence of brain damage, therefore, is concluded from the presence of hyperactivity in the child. As matters of fact, hyperactivity has been established as one possible symptom of brain damage, but not all brain damaged individuals are hyperactive, nor are all hyperactive individuals brain damaged.

The following quotations from Thomas, Chess and Birch (1968 p. 135) underscore much of what has been presented thus far on the relationship of brain damage to hyperactivity.

> The consequences of brain damage in childhood have tended to be discussed as though there regularly appears a single syndrome characterized by hyperkinesis, distractibility, perseveration, perceptual disturbance, emotional lability, atypical cognitive functioning, and disturbances in impulse control.
> ... the hyperkinetic syndrome does occur in some children as a direct consequence of central nervous system damage. At the same time, the behavioral sequelae of brain damage in childhood can be most diverse ...
> ... no pattern of behavioral dysfunction can be considered to fit all brain-damaged children.

One immediate implication of an organic theory of causation is that corrective methods should also be of an organic nature; this has led to the widespread use of drugs for controlling hyperactivity. Further detailed observations will be made in the chapter by Mira and Reece on the efficacy of medication, but the status of medication seems to be growing, not lessening, in controversy. Some critical and comprehensive reviews of the effectiveness of drug treatment include Sulzbacher (1973), a *Journal of Learning Disabilities* issue devoted to medication (1971, volume 4, number 9) and Delong (1972). Illustrations of the growing negative public response to medication are presented in three articles with the dramatic titles of "Drugging the American Child: We're too Cavalier About Hyperactivity" (Walker, 1974),

"Toward a Nation of Sedated Children" (Divoky, 1973), and "A Slavish Reliance on Drugs: Are We Pushers for Our Own Children?" (Offir, 1974).

It would be spurious indeed to conclude for or against organic factors as the main contributor to hyperactivity. Many persons accept the possibility of organic etiology; it is with specific children that it often becomes difficult to make a definitive statement. Also, organic etiology often gets expressed via the term or label *brain damage*, and there are some potential dangers connected with using the label in nonmedical settings. There is still much mystery associated with brain functioning and certainly with the notion of a damaged brain. People working with the child such as teachers or parents, if not properly oriented, could use the label as an explanation for many behaviors not really a function of the presumed damage. This could produce a sense of futility leading to an attitude of *why try anything?* Or, the label could provoke a set of erroneous behavioral expectations in teachers and parents which in turn could precipitate those behaviors. The self-fulfilling prophesy phenomenon (Rosenthal and Jacobsen, 1968) does become a very real possibility when one expects that a child will behave a certain way. The child can internalize those expectations he sees others having of him and attempt to behave accordingly.

The writer recalls meeting with a child new to the school system for purposes of a psychological study. His records had not yet arrived and there was a question as to his need for a special education program. Early in the formal testing he smiled and said, "I can't do this . . . I'm brain damaged." With some encouragement and reinforcement from the writer (an unforgivable departure from standardized procedures) he completed the task he thought he could not complete. Another child shared with the writer that his physician and mother had diagnosed him as being hyperactive and that the prescribed medication had successfully controlled his behavior. He then complained, as he sat in a relaxed, stationary fashion, that since the medication had been terminated several weeks earlier he was unable to sit still in class. His words and contradictory behavior were reminiscent of the plaintiff who demonstrated for the judge how high he was able to raise his arm before the accident.

In contrast to these illustrations of the self-fulfilling prophesy, a recent article (Schoenrade, 1974) depicted a child developing better self-understanding through the parent's explanation of how a chemical imbalance in her brain caused her to be hyperactive and required certain medication.

A number of published papers that have reviewed the literature on organic etiology (Burks, 1960; Marwitt and Stenner, 1972; Alabiso, 1972; Wender, 1971; and Werry, 1968) can offer the interested reader a more complete and technical exposure to this area, but it is interesting to note that Chess (1960) attributed only 15 percent of hyperactivity to neurological factors and that Schmitt (1974) attributed only 1 percent of hyperactivity to organic etiology.

Developmental Hyperactivity

Werry (1968), in particular, has addressed himself to the concept of developmental hyperactivity as separate from organic and psychogenic hyperactivity. His definition was cited earlier and emphasized excessive motor activity, the absence of clear evidence of brain damage or psychosis and the existence of the condition since infancy. Werry acknowledged that hyperactivity was not independent of the child's cultural background, and therefore some comparison was necessary of the child with his cultural norms.

The pattern of development described by Werry includes the child, even in infancy and early childhood, always being "on the go," attention defects, excitability, and very often, learning disorders in school. Werry's consideration of management techniques was divergent and based on his belief that the hyperactive child was also in fact multiply handicapped in terms of attention deficits, probable emotional problems and learning difficulties. His repertoire of management possibilities included medication, behavior therapy, remedial education and perceptual motor training and environmental structuring.

Related to Werry's position are the works of Kagan (1965)

on cognitive tempo and of Thomas, Chess and Birch (1968) on temperament in young children. These latter researchers identified nine categories of behavior which permitted them to establish temperament distinctions among infants and young children. The categories will briefly be described to offer the reader some idea of the scope of variables that can differentiate even infant behavior (Thomas, Chess and Birch, p. 20-24).

1. *Activity Level.* ". . . the level, tempo and frequency with which a motor component is present in the child's functioning."

2. *Rhymicity.* ". . . the degree of rhythmicity or regularity of repetitive biological functions."

3. *Approach or Withdrawal.* ". . . the child's initial reaction to any new stimulus, be it food, places, toys, or procedures."

4. *Adaptability.* ". . . the sequential course of responses a child makes to new or altered situations."

5. *Intensity of Reaction.* ". . . the energy content of the response, irrespective of its direction."

6. *Threshold of Responsiveness.* ". . . level of extrinsic stimulation that is necessary to evoke a discernible response."

7. *Quality of Mood.* ". . . the amount of pleasant, joyful, friendly behavior as contrasted with unpleasant, crying, unfriendly behavior."

8. *Distractibility.* ". . . the effectiveness of extraneous environmental stimuli in interfering with, or in altering the direction of, the ongoing behavior."

9. *Attention Span and Persistence.* ". . . the length of time a particular activity is pursued . . . the child's maintaining of an activity in the face of obstacles."

It was recognized that some children will be considerably more active, explorative and demanding than others as a function of their inborn temperament. This is not to disregard that organic factors, injuries, infections, etc., might not be contributing factors. Their work has done much to highlight just how individualistic children can be in their behavior patterns.

Kagan's (1965) work on impulsivity and reflectivity in

children is further argument for the naturally occurring differences in cognitive tempo among children. As he stated,

> Research at the Fels Institute during the past half-decade has been directed at this "decision time variable, which has been called "reflection-impulsivity." Succinctly stated, the reflection-impulsivity dimension describes the child's consistent tendency to display slow or fast response times in problem situations with high response uncertainty. The results are persuasive in suggesting that a tendency for reflection increases with age, is stable over periods as long as 20 months, manifests pervasive generality across varied task situations, and is linked to some fundamental aspects of the child's personality organization (p. 134).

In some cases the impulsivity that anxious parents or teachers observe may not have been the function of a pathological condition, but rather of the child's unique, cognitive style in action. This developmental or constitutional position raises interesting and challenging questions regarding identification of the developmental pattern, whether or not to intervene, or how to arrange the environment if direct intervention with the child is not considered.

In a comprehensive review of the literature on reflectivity-impulsivity (Epstein, Hallahan, and Kaufman, 1975) the relationship between impulsive cognitive tempo and hyperactivity was established as being quite complex. There are considerable overlaps between the two conditions, but also important differences. The lack of precision in defining hyperactivity was again identified as a confabulating factor. Those authors expressed the belief that impulsivity can be modified where school learning and adjustment were being negatively affected. They cited a variety of techniques including clear communication of teacher expectation, selective use of modeling and even the judicious use of negative feedback and punishment.

In relation to developmental hyperactivity Martin (Schmitt et al., 1973) identified three considerations that have implications for persons working with the child and his family. First, Martin felt it important for the involved persons to acknowledge that the condition may be free from brain damage or central nervous system dysfunction. Rather, the condition may be connected to an inherent biological status, or to the child's temperament, or as an entrenched personality trait. The second implication of developmental hyperactivity was its depicting of the natural variations in human behavior for which we cannot ascribe specific causes. This offers a pointed guilt-reducing message for parents. "Parents have not caused developmental hyperactivity. They have observed it and reacted to it" (Schmitt et al., 1973 p. 155).

The third and, according to Martin, the most important implication of the concept of developmental hyperactivity was the focus on helping the family and, the writer would add, teacher to adapt to the trait in the child. This is an important consideration and startling to some people in its simplicity. Rather than focussing totally on the child as needing to be changed, possibly the environment needs to be altered so as to accommodate the child.

Psychologically Derived Hyperactivity

The behavioral characteristics often associated with hyperactivity, such as short attention span, restlessness, irritability and impulsivity can easily be viewed as the manifestations of anxiety. The situational nature of hyperactivity among a number of children gives added support of the picture of a psychologically-derived hyperactivity. For example, Marwitt and Stenner (1972) delineated two patterns of hyperactivity. Their first category embodied organic, maturational and constitutional etiologies while the second category considered essentially psychological etiologies. They viewed this second category as really being *hyper-reactive* in the sense of a child reacting to inner psychological pressures (fear, anxiety) and/or to outer environmental phenomena. These authors saw this kind of hyperactivity as the learned response of the child to his experiences.

In a similar vein Friedland and Shilkret (1973) described "defensive hyperactivity" as behavior children exhibit in specific situations in some cases as a "means for keeping others at a distance and fending off the development of relationships (p. 214)." Many regular class and especially remedial reading teachers notice the progressive development of excessive physical activity, figiting and distractibility as they attempt to work closely with a youngster. The same child may appear much calmer, attentive and in control in other less demanding and threatening settings.

Additional support for this view comes from the earlier mentioned study by Kenny and his co-workers (Kenny et al., 1971). Over half of the one hundred children referred to an evaluation clinic with hyperactivity as one of the presenting complaints revealed an onset of hyperactivity at the age five or older. Reportedly many of these children were behaviorally appropriate in one-to-one situations, which could give credence to the view of their being *disturbed into hyperactivity* in certain settings or under certain conditions.

Palmer (1970) described some of the possible dynamics of psychogenic hyperactivity. He suggested that for some children when they feel bored they become more aware of their internal fears, and their subsequent excessive physical activity is an effort at *working off* the anxiety. He also saw hyperactivity as the child's means of coping with depression. In both instances the hyperactivity is a defensive, self-supporting phenomenon, but while serving one purpose for the child, it continues to defeat him in other ways such as negatively affecting school learning or peer relationships.

The picture of a stimulus-hungry child, constantly performing at a high activity level and without much forethought, was presented by Averswald (1969). This child was seen as the product of a disorganized environment wherein the child failed to acquire a sense of order. He had been unable to organize his experiences in ways that gave him a sense of identity, and he accordingly had little sense of relationships with others. Each stimulus situation would be a new experience for this child, and there would likely be an aimless, easily disorganized, impulsive quality to his behavior, with a confusion regarding how or why he felt as he did in different situations. It is through excessive motion and self-stimulation that the child would find immediate meaning in his experiences, but the child would continue to lack any sense of long-term planning or extended anticipation of future events. While Averswald was not addressing himself to hyperactive children per se, his view of how the child responds to his experiences is additive to the concept of psychologically-based hyperactivity.

Redl and Wineman's (1957) description of the breakdown of ego controls and the literature on early parenting experiences (Sigel et al., 1973; Becker, 1964; and Clausen, 1966) identified some important contributors to how children come to view themselves and how they subsequently behave. This writer's interpretation of that literature is that a hyperactive-like child has a greater probability of appearing in situations where the parents are emotionally vascillating, where a close and nurturing relationship with the child as an infant was lacking, where the parents were unable to respond supportively to the young child's dependency needs, where the parents were critical and chronically dissatisfied with the child, and where the child's aggressive behavior was directly or indirectly reinforced. A close, warm parent-child relationship characterized by acceptance of the child, the consistent application of realistic limits, and a sensitivity to the child's needs is much less likely to encourage the development of a hyperactive pattern.

Some of the data collected on families of hyperactive children would support these observations. Kenny and his co-workers (1971) reported, "Sixty-four percent of the families had evidence of major environmental pathology. Nearly one third of the children (31) lived in one-parent families or did not live with either parent. Thirty-eight of the families were considered to be overtly unstable, including history of parental institutionalization for emotional disturbance, alcoholism, drug addiction, or criminal acts. Environmental deprivation was noted in fourteen homes (p. 620)."

Stewart (1970) reported that fathers of hyperactive children often had trouble themselves in school, many were dropouts, and even as adults were noted as being restless and short-tempered. These data along with other observations were used by Stewart to support the possibility of genetically-derived inborn differences in hyperactive children. The data on fathers however also clearly says something about the parenting experiences that hyperactive children may have received.

Wunderlich (1973) made observations on how some parents, by responding to the child's hyperactive-like behavior and ignoring the child when he was behaving appropriately, may have shaped the child into a hyperactive pattern. He also identified as some possible causes of hyperactivity the child copying hyperactive models and not experiencing adequate limits.

This discussion of psychologically based hyperactivity was not meant as a blame statement against parents or teachers. It is clear that some hyperactivity is organically based, some constitutional in nature and some occurring as a function of psychological stress or faulty social learning. Few parents or teachers would knowingly want to produce or encourage a hyperactive pattern in children; yet it is possible that as a result of the organization of the environment or the nature of specific adult-child relationship patterns that hyperactivity can be fostered. This is why it becomes important in the intervention process to assess the adult-child and environment-child relationships so that potential encouragers of hyperactivity can be identified and then modified.

Because of the psychological, learned nature of the behavior those children are seen as amenable to psychotherapy and behavior manipulation. Medication is often viewed as an adjunct rather than the main form of treatment. Within the school setting the demands being made of the child should be examined to determine if they are realistic. Offering the child success experiences and the security of a more structured environment usually becomes a part of an intervention program.

Chess (1960) attributed 37 percent of hyperactivity to psychological etiology while Schmitt (1974) felt that 30 percent of hyperactivity was of a situational etiology and 9 percent of a severe psychogenic basis.

Hyperactivity and the Environment

Ruth Benedict (1934) made some observations regarding the cultural matrix within which a behavior occurs that says something about the concern of educators with hyperactivity:

One of the most striking of acts that emerge from a study of widely
varying cultures is the ease with which our abnormals function in
other cultures. It does not matter what kind of "abnormality" we
choose for illustration, those which indicate extreme instability, or
those which are more in the nature of character traits like sadism or
delusions of grandeur or persecution, there are well-defined cultures
in which these abnormals function at ease and with honor, and apparently without danger or difficulty to the society (p. 60).

Certainly the variable stimulus value attributed to hyperactivity would support the extension of Benedict's relativism to
this subject. Some home and classroom environments seem to
express a broad acceptance and accommodations of individual
differences in children while other environments are much more
circumscribed in terms of what is considered acceptable and unacceptable. The norms of one subculture or family group may
vary dramatically in certain respects from another subculture or
family group within a common community. Eisenberg (1973)
stated that:

Hyperactivity and distractibility . . . show sharp social-class association . . . In a chaotic family with no attention given to the child, the
mother has no complaints. The complaint is from the school because
the child is unable to conform. An average slum classroom white or
black, is much noisier and more active than one in a middle-class
school. Among other things, this reflects the observation that the
middle-class preschool child is probably trained in sedentary activities.
He may have had stories read to him and played games with his
parents. There are regular mealtimes when he is expected to behave
himself. All of this contrasts with the catch-as-catch can, chaotic
organization of the family with multiple problems (p. 3).

From the literature reviewed thus far there are several
observations that can be made on the interaction of the child and
the environment as it pertains to a pattern of hyperactivity. First,
there are individual differences among children as a function of
inborn biological factors. Thomas, Chess and Birch (1968) and
Kagan (1965) in particular have addressed themselves to studying these differences. Some infants and toddlers present more of a
challenge to their families because of their high activity levels,
irritability and irregularity of sleeping, eating and elimination

habits. As mothers will readily testify, some of their children were more difficult to cope with even in early infancy.

Secondly, family structures will vary in their tolerance for individual differences. This may be a function of the parents' personalities or of broader cultural factors. But this means that a *difficult* child will be accepted more readily in one family while an identical child would be viewed with dismay in another family and would become the active focus of anxious parental attention. The child is not oblivious to the impact of his behavior on his parents and their responses to him give the child important information about his adequacy and self-worth. Few children are ignorant of whether they are pleasing or disturbing their parents.

Thirdly, environments possess inherent reinforcing and shaping mechanisms that interact with the child. Excessively active, manic parents present one model for the child to imitate while reflective or methodical parents present another model. A study by Yando and Kagan (1968) demonstrated how first grade children became more reflective when placed with reflective teachers. This finding prompted those authors to suggest that it might be desirable to place extremely impulsive boys with teachers who are temperamentally reflective because of the potential for the boys to become more reflective.

The fourth observation is that for many children school becomes a new psychological situation. This concept has been discussed in detail by Myerson (1963) in relation to the physically disabled person, but it certainly has application to the hyperactive child. As a product of the interaction of his unique behavioral proclivities with the home environment, the child enters the classroom, possibly to face a set of drastically different environmental forces. For some children their home experiences, parental values, expectations, etc., correlated highly with the classroom, but for other children it will be almost a totally new psychological experience. Children who are out of step with the classroom values and behavioral guidelines are going to have to change or likely be labelled as deviant. Any classroom environment (a) will vary in its acceptance and rejection of certain child behaviors, (b) will identify certain child behaviors as deviant and (c) will directly and indirectly reinforce certain behaviors. The teacher, of course, is central to these three classroom phenomenon, which is why we can find an identical set of child behaviors being accepted in one classroom and the target of much teacher concern in the next classroom.

It is apparent that the hyperactive child, if viewed from a disease or deficiency viewpoint, becomes the locus of the problem. The problem is believed to be centered in the child and the diagnostic and treatment considerations will likely focus primarily, if not totally, on the child. But if the child is viewed as one component of a system, then since each system component is interrelated, the locus of the problem shifts from the child to the system. This does not mean that all etiological considerations are separated from the child, but rather it is recognized that it is child-based variables in interaction with system-based variables that produce the problem. Rhodes (1968, 1970) in particular has contributed to the literature on how environmental factors can participate in the establishing and maintenance of "problem behavior." The implications for education are clear. "Don't just look at the child; look at the environment within which the behavior is occurring." Attempts to improve a problem situation may require that attention be directed to the child, to the teacher, to the instructional process, to the classroom physical structure, or to all of these factors.

HOW CAN WE INTERVENE?

Hyperactive children as a group can generally be distinguished from a normal sample of children, but once we examine a group of hyperactive children, a number of differences of cognitive, emotional and sensory-motor nature become evident among children.

No two hyperactive children are the same in any respect. Neither the degrees of distractibility nor the relationship between characteristics of psychopathology is ever identical in these children. In one child the problem may be chiefly visuo-motor; in a second, predominantly audio-motor; in a third, hyperkinesis and tactuo-motor. The concept of a group of hyperactive children is a figment of someone's imagination, for groups of children with sufficiently homogeneous characteristics to be considered comparable for educational purposes do not exist.

(Cruickshank, 1967 p. 61)

These individual differences hold important implications for intervention programs. The subsequent chapters will address themselves in total or in part with intervention procedures for hyperactive children. The purpose of this section is to offer the reader an overview of orientations, beliefs and methods of intervention. Also, some strategies and assumptions will be presented here that will not be covered elsewhere.

The decision to intervene with a hyperactive child leads to a number of judgments about how to help that child. Any program that is systematic in nature will consider the purposes or goals of the intervention, the focus of the intervention, the kinds of procedures and the personnel involved.

Purposes of the Intervention

What do we hope to accomplish as a result of intervention? If we accept that hyperactive children differ from each other, then it becomes necessary to decide on what changes we want to occur for each child. The following is a listing of some possible objectives. Each of these statements could be reduced even further and expressed as narrow behavioral objectives:

a. to increase school learning (or learning in a specific subject; or the acquisition of very specific subject processes, such as carrying in two-column addition)
b. to decrease excessive physical activity
c. to decrease the child's disruptiveness
d. to improve the self-concept
e. to improve peer relationships
f. to improve specific motor skills
g. to improve social skills

The advantages of further reducing these statements to narrow behavioral objectives is that we become even clearer in our goals. Also, the attainment of those goals becomes more easily measurable. If, for example, *improved social skills* could be subdivided into specific observable behaviors such as *play cooperatively with another child* or *reduction in number of arguments,* then we could both measure the behaviors more easily and define and evaluate a program calculated to achieve those goals.

Focus of the Intervention

We ought not assume that the intervention procedures will necessarily be applied directly to the child. While our final objectives often will relate to changes in the child, the specific procedures may well focus elsewhere. We may elect to work with the peer group or the teacher regarding their attitudes and behavior toward the hyperactive child. The curriculum either in its content or in the way it is structured may become the focus of concern. Also, the instructional environment such as regular class versus special class or physical changes in the class may become the variable that is manipulated.

The focus of the intervention accordingly may be one or a combination of the following:

a. the hyperactive child
b. the peer group
c. the teacher
d. the content of the curriculum
e. the structure of the curriculum
f. the instructional environment

Personnel Involved

Some intervention procedures such as drugs automatically require a certain person—the physician—but other intervention strategies may permit options regarding the personnel involved. For example, the strategy of sensory-motor training may involve the classroom teacher, a physical education teacher, the school nurse, the psychologist or a learning disabilities consultant. Any of these persons might have or could acquire the technical skills necessary to work with the child, presuming that there was a structured program to follow.

The child himself may be the key person involved if the intervention strategy is some self-monitoring process such as the child keeping track of his academic output or the number of times out-of-seat. Possibly some of the child's classmates would assume certain observer responsibilities, or some paraprofessionals (parents, teacher aides, etc.) could be used.

The following is a listing of many of the personnel that could be involved in implementing an intervention strategy. This is not meant to detract from a current emphasis on *team* approach but simply to identify some logical human resources.

a. the classroom teacher
b. the hyperactive child
c. classroom peers
d. the physician
e. the school psychologist
f. the school nurse
g. the L.D. consultant
h. paraprofessionals

Specific Intervention Strategies

There has been no shortage in the literature of proposals for treating hyperactive children. The lack of agreement on etiology in conjunction with the prevalence and seriousness of hyperactivity has stimulated much thinking on intervention. Actual data testifying to the effectiveness of a procedure has been more difficult to come by than conjecture. For example, Pulaski (1974) found that physically active children were low in fantasy. While her research was not concerned with hyperactive children per se, she commented that possibly training hyperactive children to develop fantasy would be a means of helping them to sit still and concentrate. This interesting observation is one more example of the kind of conjecturing that exists with hyperactive children.

The following is an identification and brief discussion of several possible intervention strategies on which there is some documentation.

Medication

Certainly the most widespread method of treating hyperactive children is through medication. While numerous children have been helped, there is evidence of abuse or at least questionable management of a drug regime. Aside from periodic sensationalistic articles on the "drugging of children," there have been some recent professional articles that have brought the use and effectiveness of drug therapy into focus (DeLong 1972 and Sulzbacher, 1972). ". . . without exercising sustained caution about the influence of procedural biases on the results of studies of the effect of psychotropic medication on children, the practitioner will not find the existing research literature useful or an adequate base from which to make valid judgments about using pharmacologic approaches to learning and behavior disorders in children" (Sulzbacher, 1973 p. 516).

One of the greatest failures in drug treatment is in proper monitoring of its effects on the child. Often school personnel are unaware that the child has been placed on medication. While on one hand this might control for a *placebo effect,* the physician is often left without meaningful classroom data on which to make his judgment regarding the effects of the medication and the need to regulate dosage.

Bosco (1975) reported on studies showing a highly favorable attitude by teachers toward the use of stimulant drugs such as Ritalin.® Administrators' attitudes, however, were decidedly negative. This difference in attitude may reflect the good judgment of administrators and the desperation of teachers who were willing to accept any procedure that promised to manage the behavior of the excessively active child. The article by Bosco (1975) included several specific recommendations for educators that seem quite valuable:

1. Some states have enacted legislation regulating the behavior of teachers and other educational personnel in drug treatment programs. These laws may concern the storage and administration of drugs within public schools. School system administrators should communicate and interpret these laws to teachers.
2. Teachers should avoid such statements as, "I think Billy's work and behavior would benefit if he took Ritalin." Teachers are not qualified

to make such judgments; in order for a physician to make a proper diagnosis, a careful and thorough examination is necessary.

3. The decision to recommend medical consultation should not be made until there is reasonable assurance that the child's problem does not stem from inadequacies in the teacher or other aspects of the school environment. Drug therapy is not appropriate when the cause of the problem is boredom or inappropriate standards set by teachers.

4. Physicians who issue prescriptions for stimulant drugs on the basis of a brief interview with a parent and a cursory examination should be avoided when there is suspicion of hyperkinesis. Certainly no school official should channel parents to physicians who simply ratify the teacher's diagnosis and prescription. Many communities have physicians who specialize in the treatment of learning and behavior problems of children. Such persons are most likely to provide proper treatment.

5. Educators and physicians should collaborate in the development of monitoring systems for children being treated with drugs because of learning and behavior disorders. There are many differences between physicians and teachers in language and perspective. Thus there is little reason to expect that interprofessional communication will be easy. In some communities instruments for providing information from the teacher have been standardized. The effective treatment of learning disorders with drugs requires an unprecedented level of coordination between physicians and teachers. School officials can begin the process of communication leading toward coordination by requesting an opportunity to meet with physicians in staff meetings held within the local hospital or in meetings of specialists (e.g. pediatricians).

6. School system administrators should be aware of the numbers of children who are being advised by the school to seek medical treatment for learning-related problems. School or classrooms with unusually high referral rates should be investigated to determine if the school personnel are overly reliant on the use of drugs to solve classroom problems (pp. 491-492).

Behavior Modification

The following overview statements on behavior modification were presented in an earlier publication (Fine, 1973 pp. 3-4) :

The term behavior modification has been used to describe any systematic and operationalized procedure calculated to modify the behavior of an individual. However, the theoretical roots of the more common procedures come from conditioning and stimulus-response learning theories, with emphasis on the measurement and manipulation of observable behaviors. The specific techniques typically focus on altering the events that precede or follow the behavior as opposed to concern with such intervening variables as the person's self concept or psychological needs. For example, one popular behavior modification approach requires the teacher to first identify or pinpoint a specific behavior that needs to be changed, either increased or decreased. Next, the teacher would observe the behavior and record its current frequency or duration of occurrence. Then the teacher would change either some preceding event to the behavior such as number of mathematics problems presented or the child's seating arrangement, or some consequent event to the behavior such as selectively ignoring or rewarding the behavior. The teacher would continue to observe and evaluate the effects of this change on the child's behavior. It is important that the behaviors selected for modification be clearly defined, that only one or two be worked on at a time, and that the occurrence of the behavior be accurately observed. It is assumed that the behavior is being either triggered off by the preceding events or somehow reinforced by events following the behavior.

Over the last decade the behavioral viewpoint has become one of the most dominant forces in education. The emphasis has been decidedly on ignoring the presumed biological or psychodynamic causes of behavior and focussing instead on the observable behaviors. A number of relevant studies have been reported that would encourage considering behavior modification techniques with hyperactive children. These studies have included preschoolers as well as older children and even whole classrooms (Allen, Henke, Harris, Baer and Reynolds, 1967; Patterson, Jones, Whittier, and Wright, 1965; McKenzie, Clark, Wolf, Kothera and Benson, 1968; and Vance, 1969).

An interesting variation on the traditional reinforcement theme was reported by Nixon (1969). In this study social modeling procedures were used which involved showing the hyperactive children short film scenarios of task-oriented and distractible, hyperactive behaviors. The assumption, seemingly an apt one for young hyperactive children, was that many of these children probably were unaware of the differences between on-task and hyperactive behaviors. The children were tangibly and immediately reinforced for discriminating the behaviors being observed. Once it was established that the children could discriminate among behaviors, reinforcement procedures were then applied directly to the actual classroom behaviors of the children.

A recent well-designed study demonstrated that hyperactivity could be controlled through the reinforcement of academic performance (Allyon, Laymann, and Kandel, 1975). In the absence of the formerly controlling medication that the three children had been receiving and in the presence of reinforcement for solely academic performance, the children both increased their academic performance and decreased their hyperactivity.

Another theme in behavior modification is the involvement of the child in programs of self-management. This can vary from the child deciding on the behaviors to change to the child selecting the immediate and back-up reinforcers and even the schedule of reinforcement. Where hyperactivity is part of a pattern of marked personality disorganization, it may not be realistic to offer the child much decision making. In cases where the child is reasonably intact intellectually and emotionally he may respond enthusiastically to participating in his own intervention program.

The chapter by Herbert Rieth treats this area in detail, describing variations in measurement and reinforcement procedures.

Dietary Management

A recent book by Feingold (1975) presented an argument for the relationship between diet and hyperactivity. The author, an allergist and pediatrician, described how some individuals can be affected behaviorally by certain common foods and the chemicals found in many food additives. The data he shared was primarily of a case study nature without rigorous scientific control, but he did identify some current studies of a controlled nature that are testing his hypotheses. Feingold referred to a major study directed by Dr. Keith Conners and funded by the National Institute of Education.

Diet and allergy as possible causal factors of hyperactivity have been discussed by other writers. Wunderlich (1970 pp. 300-

301) stated "Many hyperkinetic children are allergic children by virtue of clinical history or by physical examination of the nasal mucous membranes. It is wise to remember that oranges, chocolate, egg, wheat, or milk can be directly responsible for hyperactive behavior. There is nothing more tragic than the untreated allergic hyperactive, for proper allergic management will often result in disappearance of the hyperactivity!"

There seems little question or controversy with the notion that a diet or allergy viewpoint has something to contribute to our understanding of the cause and management (or even cure) of hyperactivity. Controversy does exist between those who would argue that most hyperactivity can be accounted for via this view and those who believe only a small percentage of hyperactive children are affected by diet.

Fortunately, more scientifically derived data seem to be on the way to clarify this question.

Cognitive Self-Management

The nature of an impulsive act is that there is little forethought involved. From this assumption, some researchers have felt that hyperactive or impulsive children might be able to more adequately monitor their behavior if they learned to talk to themselves in certain ways. There have been reports of success with variations of self-instructions (Bem, 1967; Palkes, Stewart, and Kahana, 1972; and Meichenbaum and Goodman, 1971).

The use of such procedures was overviewed in a recent article by Meichenbaum and Cameron (1974). One of the procedures used had a model (this could be a teacher or remedial educator) verbalizing instructions to the child, then had the child repeat and act out the instructions. The writer observed a similar procedure being applied with a hyperactive child in a remedial education situation. The child typically worked excessively quickly, ignoring parts of math problems. He was verbally instructed by the remedial teacher to "Look at each problem carefully and decide what you are supposed to do. Take your time and think about each question. Then begin." The child orally repeated the instructions and proceeded to the problems. These self-directions were subsequently written out and the child read them aloud before starting each new problem. As would be expected, satiation is a hazard with this kind of procedure. Another important consideration is the eventual fading of the self-instructual procedures so that the child functions more normally in the classroom.

Meichenbaum and Cameron presented some optimistic data and some suggestions that should stimulate additional research and demonstration. For example, they have had the impulsive child practice giving verbal directions to another person on how to perform a task; they have also experimented with impulsive children teaching a younger child how to do a task.

Learning Body Control

The hyperactive child has been described as experiencing a lack of awareness of his body actions. The child may be sitting at his desk trying to concentrate, but with his legs, feet, hands and fingers moving constantly and erratically. When the children are instructed to line up, the child may continue to move his feet, stepping forward and backward, bumping into other children. The teacher's sharp admonition to "Stand still!" may be met by a bewildered look from the child who is unaware of what he has been doing motorically.

Accordingly, some researchers have advocated the use of procedures that would increase the child's awareness of his motor behavior. These procedures have been described under different labels such as *relaxation training, biofeedback techniques, breathing control* and simply *increasing body awareness*. It is not uncommon to find several procedures incorporated into a program. For example, in a study reported by Simpson and Nelson (1974) the goal was to help a group of hyperactive children develop self-control over motor behavior and to maintain attention in some specified learning situations. The children were trained in breathing patterns utilizing biofeedback procedures so they would be aware of how they were breathing; also the children received reinforcement following their maintaining a particular breathing pattern. The results of this study were somewhat mixed but encouraging of further research.

Jacobson (1973) categorized many of the behaviors that are characteristic of hyperactive children as signs of overtension, "What then are common signs of overtension in pupils? Overaction is one, restlessness, another, failure to sit still and to stand still; rapid movements, even when inappropriate; rapid speech, sometimes inarticulate (p. 57)."

Jacobson's proposed solution was a program of systematic relaxation, and in his book he presents a detailed set of procedures that teachers can use with children of different ages.

Another easy-to-follow set of directions for relaxation training was offered by Koeppen (1974). Her relaxation training script moves the children sequentially through specific body parts, requiring first tensing, then relaxing. The language seems appropriate for young children, and her directions are very explicit. For example, in relation to the jaw, she instructs the children as follows:

> You have a giant jawbreaker bubble gum in your mouth. It's very hard to chew. Bite down on it. Hard! Let your neck muscles help you. Now relax. Just let your jaw hang loose. Notice how good it feels just to let your jaw drop. Okay, let's tackle that jawbreaker again now. Bite down. Hard! Try to squeeze it out between your teeth. That's good. You're really tearing that gum up. Now relax again. Just let your jaw drop off your face. It feels so good just to let go and not have to fight that bubble gum. Okay, one more time. We're really going to tear it up this time. Bite down. Hard as you can. Harder. Oh, you're really working hard. Good. Now relax. Try to relax your whole body. You've beaten the bubble gum. Let yourself go as loose as you can (p. 18).

The results of biofeedback procedures have been limited and mixed. A recent study (Braud, Lupin, and Braud, 1975) using a single six-year-old hyperactive boy reported desirable changes along several dimensions including muscle tension reduction, parent and teacher behavior ratings, and achievement gains. The research reported by Nall (1973) on the use of alpha biofeedback procedures had different results. Three groups were utilized in one of the studies, a training group, a placebo group and a control group. There were no significant differences among the three groups following approximately three months of twenty minutes per day training. The variables assessed included hyperkinetic and maladaptive behavior, academic achievement and even the ability to produce Alpha waves.

The teaching of body control, under its various labels, seems to hold some promise for hyperactive children. It is a new area of study that is based on some exciting theorizing despite the absence of extensive supportive data. One obvious advantage is that it is an alternative to medication. Also, it is the child's increased self-awareness and self-control that are the important goals of body control training rather than simply reinforced behavior changes.

Instructional Designs

The teacher's pragmatic questions on how to teach the hyperactive child have clearly not been answered. Medication, autoinstructions, behavior modification, modelling techniques and, presumably, diet management have all contributed to a relatively more manageable child, but the literature fails to support a universally effective procedure for instructional design.

It is probably more realistic and functional to consider the educational needs of each individual child rather than generalizing to all hyperactive children. This was basically the opinion of Forness (1975, p. 160) who stated,

> . . . each hyperactive child should be dealt with according to his or her own level of readiness for regular classroom functioning. Options would range from full-time placement in a special class to enrollment in a regular classroom with supportive assistance to the child's teacher. The fact that a child is hyperactive does not necessarily preordain him to a particular approach. Curriculum materials and techniques developed with mentally retarded children or children with sensory defects have, in fact, been effectively applied to children labeled hyperactive and vice versa.

Generalizations have occurred regarding the educational needs of hyperactive children. The writings of the early *minimal brain damage* theorists (Strauss and Lehtinen, 1947; Strauss and Kephart, 1955; Cruickshank, Bentzen, Ratzeburg and Tannhauser, 1961; and Cruickshank, 1967) proposed that the hyperactive child could not properly organize many stimuli and that this led to excessive and disorganized reactivity. The logical instructional design seemed to be a destimulated environment. For example, children were taught in cubicles that controlled visual stimuli. Dull colors were advocated for the physical surroundings as well as acoustical wall and ceiling materials to reduce the noise level. Zentell (1975) refers to this approach as a "stimulus reduction theory." As was mentioned earlier, there is limited empirical support for this view. Actually a number of studies have seriously questioned the efficacy of a stimulus-reduced environment (Somervill, Warnberg, and Bost, 1973; Rost and Charles, 1967; and Shores and Havbrich, 1969). The one major study reported by proponents of the approach (Cruickshank, Bentzen, Ratzeburg and Tannhauser, 1971) was in fact inconclusive. However, the study represented a rich description of classroom procedures and specific teaching techniques.

Zentell (1975), through a selective review of the literature, presents the argument that the hyperactive child may actually be seeking greater stimulation; he suggests that many of the classic descriptors of hyperactivity (inattentiveness, impulsivity, distractibility) actually decrease under conditions of increased sensory stimulation.

The instructional strategies advocated by Frank Hewitt (1968) have led to an "engineered environment" where all of the child's experiences are monitored. This approach embodies the basic principles of behavior modification and task analysis. The child is trained in prelearning skills such as listening and following directions, then is systematically subjected to simple instructional demands. The child's progress is constantly monitored and the child then progresses through a learning sequence involving modifications of imposed structure until he is ready to return to a regular classroom setting. There has been some empirical support for Hewitt's approach (Hewitt, 1972).

In relation to instructional procedures a potentially helpful collection of classroom activities has been compiled by Connor (1974), but once again it remains with the teacher's sensitivity to individual pupil need as to when and how to utilize the specific procedures.

A considerably more extensive review of educational procedures is offered in Norma Dyck's chapter, which also includes a more detailed description of the approaches advocated by Cruickshank and Hewitt.

SUMMARY

Hyperactive children have been around for some time and have received much attention from many different disciplines. Indeed these children seem to have served almost as a projective test for experts who all see evidence to support their notions on etiology and management.

Concensus does exist on a number of facets of the hyperactive child such as the salient characteristics and the likelihood that there may be several interacting causal factors, but in many ways this child remains enigmatic and troublesome for parents, educators and others concerned with the child's welfare. Even after the more visible symptoms have decreased, usually by puberty, the child is often left with such residuals as lower academic achievement and poor self-concept.

The major efforts at treatment or management have focussed quite behaviorally on symptom reduction, usually through behavior modification, destimulating the environment or medication. Very little is reported in the literature on assisting the child toward greater self-awareness and increased capacity for self-management.

The literature is encouraging from several viewpoints. First, there seems to be an increase of articles, studies and books, all testifying to a desirable growing professional interest in the area. Secondly, the literature is productive in presenting empirically-based programs and methodologies for working with hyperactive children. And, thirdly, the literature reflects a broad attack on the problems of hyperactivity, including diet management, biofeedback procedures, sensory-motor training and cognitive self-management.

REFERENCES

Alabiso, F.: Inhibitory functions of attention in reducing hyperactive behavior. *Am J Ment Defic, 77*:259-282, 1972.

Allen, K. E., Henke, L. B., Harris, F. R., Baier, D. M., and Reynolds, N. J.: Control of hyperactivity by social reinforcement of attending behaviors. *J Ed Psychol, 56*:231-237, 1967.

Allyon, T., Layman, D., and Kandel, H. J.: A behavioral-educational alternative to drug control of hyperactive children. *J Appl Beh Anal, 8*:137-146, 1975.

Averswald, E. H.: Cognitive development and psychopathology in the urban environment. In Graubard, P. S. (Ed.): *Children Against the Schools*. Chicago, Follett, 1969.

Becker, W. C.: Consequences of different kinds of parental discipline. In Hoffman, L. W., and Hoffman, M. L. (Eds.): *Review of Child Development Research*. New York, Russell Sage Foundation, 1964, vol. 1.

Bem, S.: Verbal self-control: The establishment of effective self-instruction. *J Exp Psychol, 74*:485-491, 1967.

Benedict, R.: Anthropology and the abnormal. *J Gen Psychol, 10*:59-80, 1934.

Bosco, J.: Behavior modification drugs and the schools: The case of Ritalin. *Phi Delta Kappan, 56*:489-492, 1975.

Braud, L. W., Lupin, M. N., and Braud, W. G.: The use of electromyographic biofeedback in the control of hyperactivity. *J Learn Disabil, 8*:420-425, 1975.

Buddenhagen, R. G., and Sickler, P.: Hyperactivity: A forty-eight hour sample plus a note on etiology. *Am J Ment Defic, 27*:580-589, 1969.

Burks, H. F.: The hyperkinetic child, *Except Child, 27*:18-26, 1960.

Chess, S.: Diagnosis and treatment of the hyperactive child. *NY State J Med, 60*:2379-2385, 1960.

Clausen, J. A.: Family structure, socialization, and personality. In Hoffman, L. W., and Hoffman, M. L. (Eds.): *Review of Child Development Research*. New York, Russell Sage Foundation, vol. 2, 1966.

Conner, J. P.: *Classroom Activities for Helping Hyperactive Children*. New York, The Center for Applied Research in Education, 1974.

Conners, C. K.: Psychological assessment of children with minimal brain dysfunction. *Ann NY Acad Sci, 205*:283-302, 1973.

Cruickshank, W. M.: Hyperactive children: Their needs and curriculum. In Knoblock, P., and Johnson, J. L. (Eds.): *The Teaching-Learning Pro-*

cess in Educating Emotionally Disturbed Children. Syracuse, Syracuse U Pr, 1967.

Cruickshank, W. M., Bentzen, F. A., Ratzeburg, F., and Tannhauser, M. T.: *A Teaching Method for Brain-Injured and Hyperactive Children.* Syracuse, Syracuse U Pr, 1961.

DeLong, A. R.: What have we learned from psychoactive drug research on hyperactives? *Am J Dis Child, 123*:177-180, 1972.

Divoky, D.: Toward a nation of sedated children. *Learning, 1*:6-13, 1973.

Doulgas, V.: Stop, look and listen: The problem of sustained attention and impulse control in hyperactive and normal children. *Can J Beh Sci, 4*:259-282, 1972.

Ebaugh, F. G.: Neuropsychiatric sequelae of acute epidemic encephalitis in children. *Am J Dis Child, 25*:89-97, 1923.

Eisenberg, L.: The overactive child. *Hosp Practice, 8*:1-10, 1973.

Emblem, D. L.: For a disciplinarians manual. *Phi Delta Kappan, 50*:339-340, 1969.

Epstein, M. H., Hallahan, D. P., and Kaufman, J. M.: Implications of the reflectivity-impulsivity dimension for special education. *J Spec Ed, 9*:11-25, 1975.

Feingold, B. F.: *Why Your Child Is Hyperactive.* New York, Random, 1975.

Fine, M.J.: *The Teacher's Role in Classroom Management.* Lawrence, Kansas, Psych-Ed Associates, 1973.

Forness, S.: Educational approaches with hyperactive children. In Cantwell, D. P. (Ed.): *The Hyperactive Child.* Holliswood, Spectrum Publications, 1975.

Freibergs, V., and Douglas, V.: Concept learning in hyperactive and normal children. *J Abnorm Psychol, 74*:388-395, 1969.

Friedland, S. J., and Shilkret, R. B.: Alternative explanations of learning disabilities: Defensive hyperactivity. *Except Child, 40*:213-215, 1973.

Hewett, F. M.: *The Emotionally Disturbed Child in the Classroom.* Boston, Allyn, 1968.

Hewett, F.: Educational programs for children with behavior disorders. In Quay, H., and Werry, J. (Eds.): *Psychopathological Disorders of Childhood.* New York, Wiley, 1972.

Horenstein, S. R.: Resperine and chlorpromazine in hyperactive mental defectives. *Am J Ment Defic, 61*:525-529, 1957.

Huessy, H. R.: Study of the prevalence and therapy of the choreatiform syndrome or hyperkinesis in rural Vermont. *Acta Paedopsychiatry, 34*:130-135, 1967.

Jacobson, E.: *Teaching and Learning.* Chicago, National Foundation for Progressive Relaxation, 1973.

Kagan, J.: Impulsive and reflective children: Significance of conceptual tempo. In Krumboltz, J. D. (Ed.): *Learning and the Educational Process.* Chicago, Rand McNally, 1965.

44   INTERVENTION WITH HYPERACTIVE CHILDREN

Kahn, E., and Cohen, L. H.: Organic driveness — a brain stem syndrome and an experience — with case reports. N Engl J Med, 210:748-756, 1934.

Kenny, T. J., Clemmens, R. L., Hudson, B. W., Lentz, G. A., Cicci, R., and Nair, P.: Characteristics of children referred because of hyperactivity. J Dediatr, 79:618-622, 1971.

Keogh, B. K., Tchir, C., and Windeguth-Behn, A.: Teachers' perceptions of educationally high risk children. J Learn Disabil, 7:43-50, 1974.

Keogh, B.: Hyperactivity and learning disorders: Review and speculation. Except Child, 38:101-109, 1971.

Koeppen, A. S.: Relaxation training for children. Elementary School Guidance and Counseling, 9:14-21, 1974.

Laufer, M. W.: Cerebral dysfunction and behavior disorders in adolescents. Am J Orthopsychiatry, 32:501-506, 1962.

Laufer, M. W.: Brain disorders. In Freedman, A. M., and Kaplan, H. I. (Ed.): The Child: His Psychological and Cultural Development. New York, Atheneum, 1972, vol. 2.

Loney, J.: The intellectual functioning of hyperactive elementary school boys: a cross sectional investigation. Am J Orthopsychiatry, 44:754-762, 1974.

Marwitt, S. J., and Stenner, A. J.: Hyperkinesis: Delineation of two patterns. Except Child, 38:401-406, 1972.

Mauer, A.: Corporal punishment. Am Psychol, 29:614-626, 1974.

McIntosh, D. K., and Dunn, L. M.: Children with specific learning disabilities. In Dunn, L. M. (Ed.): Exceptional Children in the Schools, 2nd Edition. New York, HR & W, 1973.

McKenzie, H. S., Clark, M., Wolf, M. M., Kethera, R., and Benson, C.: Behavior modification of children with learning disabilities using grades as tokens and allowances as back up reinforcers. Except Child, 34:745-752, 1968.

Meichenbaum, D., and Goodman, J.: Training impulsive children to talk to themselves: A means of developing self control. J Abnorm Psychol, 77: 115-126, 1971.

Meichenbaum, D., and Cameron, R.: The clinical potential of modifying what clients say to themselves. Psychotherapy: Theory, Research and Practice, 11:103-117, 1974.

Menkes, M. M., Rowe, J. S., and Menkes, J. H.: A twenty-five year followup study on the hyperkinetic child with minimal brain dysfunction. Pediatrics, 39:393-399, 1967.

Minde, K., Lewin, D., Weiss, G., Lavigueur, H., Douglas, V., and Sykes, E.: The hyperactive child in elementary school: A five year, controlled follow-up. Except Child, 38:214-221, 1971.

Myerson, L.: Somatopsychology of physical disability. In Cruickshank, W. (Ed.): Psychology of Exceptional Children and Youth, 2nd Edition. Englewood Cliffs, P-H, 1963.

Nall, A.: Alpha training and the hyperkinetic child . . . is it effective? *Acad Ther, 9:*5-19, 1973.

Nixon, S. B.: Increasing task-oriented behavior. In Krumboltz, J. D., and Thoreson, C. E. (Ed.): *Behavioral Counseling.* New York, HR & W, 1969.

Offir, C. W.: A slavish reliance on drugs; Are we pushers for our own children? *Psychol Today, 8:*49, 1974.

Palkes, H., Stewart, M., and Freedman, J.: Improvement in maze performance of hyperactive boys as a function of verbal-training procedures. *J Spec Ed, 5:*337-342, 1972.

Palmer, J. O.: *The Psychological Assessment of Children.* New York, Wiley, 1970.

Paraskevopoulos, J., and McCarthy, J.: Behavior patterns of children with special learning disabilities. *Psychol Schools, 7:*42-46, 1970.

Patterson, G. R., Hones, R., Whittier, J., and Wright, M. A.: A behavior modification technique for the hyperactive child. *Beh Res Ther, 2:*217-226, 1965.

Pulaski, M. A.: The rich rewards of make believe. *Psychol Today, 7:*68-74, 1974.

Redl, F., and Wineman, D.: *The Aggressive Child.* New York, Free Pr, 1957.

Rhodes, W.: The disturbing child: A problem of ecological management. *Except Child, 33:*449-455, 1967.

Rhodes, W.: A community participation analysis of emotional disturbance. *Except Child, 36:*309-314, 1970.

Rogers, M. E., Lilienfeld, A. M., and Pasamanick, B.: Prenatal and paranatal factors in the development of childhood behavior disorders. *Acta Psychiatrica Scandinavica, 1:*1-157, (Suppl. 102), 1955.

Rosenthal, R., and Jacobson, L.: *Pygmalion in the classroom.* New York, HR & W, 1968.

Rost, K. J., and Charles, D. C.: Academic achievement of brain injured and hyperactive children in isolation. *Except Child, 34:*125-126, 1967.

Schmitt, B. D.: The hyperactive child. Paper presented at the University of Kansas Medical Center, Kansas City, June, 1974.

Schmitt, B. D., Martin, H. P., Nellhaus, G., Cravens, J., Camp, B. W., and Jordan, K.: The hyperactive child. *Clin Pediatr, 12:*154-169, 1973.

Schoenrade, J. L.: Help means hope for Laurie. *J Learn Disabil, 7:*23-25, 1974.

Schrager, J., Lindy, J., Harrison, S., McDermott, J., and Killins, E.: The hyperkinetic child: Some consensually validated behavioral correlates. *Except Child, 32:*635-637, 1966.

Shores, R. E., and Havbrich, P. A.: Effect of cubicles in educating emotionally disturbed children. *Except Child, 36:*21-24, 1969.

Sigel, I. E., Starr, R., Secrist, A., Jackson, J. P., and Hill, E.: Social and emotional development of young children. In Frost, J. L. (Ed.): *Revisit-*

ing *Early Childhood Education.* New York, HR & W 1973. Originally printed in Grotberg, E. (Ed.): *Day Care: Resources for Decisions.* Washington, OEO, 1971.

Simpson, D. D., and Nelson, A. E.: Attention training through breathing control to modify hyperactivity. *J Learn Disabil, 7:*274-283, 1974.

Solomons, G.: The hyperactive child. *J Iowa Med Soc, 55:*464-469, 1965.

Solomons, G.: Guidelines on the use and medical effects of psychostimuland drugs in therapy. *J Learn Disabil, 9:*470-475, 1971.

Somervill, J. W., Warnberg, L. S., and Bost, D. E.: Effects of cubicles versus increased stimulation on task performance by first-grade males perceived as distractible and nondistractible. *J Spec Ed, 7:*169-185, 1970.

Stewart, M. A., and Olds, S. W.: *Raising a Hyperactive Child.* New York, Harper and Row, 1973.

Stewart, M. A.: Hyperactive children. *Sci Am, 222:*94-99, 1970.

Stewart, M. A., Pitts, F. N., Craig, A. G., and Dieruf, W.: The hyperactive child syndrome. *Am J Orthopsychiatry, 36:*861-867, 1966.

Strauss, A. A., and Lehtinen, L. E.: *Psychopathology and Education of the Brain-Injured Child.* New York, Grune, 1947.

Strauss, A. A., and Kephart, N. C.: *Psychopathology and Education of the Brain-Injured Child, II.* New York, Grune, 1955.

Sulzbacher, S. I.: Psychotropic medication with children: An evaluation of procedural biases in results of reported studies. *Pediatrics, 51:*513-517, 1973.

Thomas, A., Chess, S., and Birch, H. G.: *Temperament and Behavior Disorders in Children.* New York, New York U Pr, 1968.

Vance, B.: Modifying hyperactive and aggressive behavior. In Krumboltz, J. D., and Thoresen, C. E. (Ed.): *Behavioral Counseling.* New York, HR & W, 1969.

Walker, S.: Drugging the American child: We're too cavalier about hyperactivity. *Psychol Today, 8:*43-48, 1974.

Wender, P. H.: *Minimal Brain Dysfunction in Children.* New York, Wiley-Interscience, 1971.

Werry, J. S.: Developmental hyperactivity. *Pediatr Clin North Am, 15:*581-599, 1968.

Wunderlich, R. C.: *Kids, Brains, and Learning.* St. Petersburg, Johnny Reads, 1970.

Wunderlich, R. C.: Treatment of the hyperactive child. *Acad Ther, 8:*375-390, 1973.

Yando, R., and Kagan, J.: The effect of teacher tempo on the child. *Child Devel, 39:*27-34, 1968.

2

Medical management of the hyperactive child

Mary Mira and Carol Ann Reece

INTRODUCTION

IN THIS CHAPTER we will present a description
of the optimal program of medical management of hyperactive children and the rationale for such a program. We do not present this as a treatment option that one might select in lieu of another type of treatment, but rather as a program which articulates with other management regimes in home and school, and which is a necessary part of the treatment of any hyperactive child. We present this so that school personnel, particularly school psychologists, have the information to make full and appropriate use of medical services and to assess the care that the child is receiving.

It is vital that school personnel be sophisticated about pediatric care of children with behavioral disabilities, particularly hyperactive children, since the school is a major channel to the physician's office for these children. The teacher is often the first person to talk openly about the abnormality of a child's behavior. In a survey of teacher practices with respect to hyperactive children

Robin and Bosco (1973) found that 40 percent of their respond-
ents indicated that when they had a child with a behavior problem
in class they suggested to parents that the child be taken to his
doctor. In a survey of children referred to a medical center clinic
because of *hyperactivity*, Kenny et al. (1971) found that over half
were referred directly by a school system.

Before outlining what we feel is the best program given what
is known about hyperactivity at the present time, we would like to
describe the general attitude about hyperactive children as we see
it in our referrals and the messages that this attitude conveys about
how we are expected to evaluate and treat them.

A POPULAR VIEW OF HYPERACTIVITY

One component of this attitude is the view that the behavior
of these children represents a chronic, long-standing pattern of
problem behavior with remote origins beyond the classroom,
that the behavior is deviant and a problem to the environment.
The school views the behavior as negative in that it is disruptive
to the efficient management of a classroom and it interferes with
the child's own progress through the academic curriculum as well
as with the development of his social skills. Those parents who
have tuned in to the child's behavior in the toddler years, although they may not have made persistent efforts to seek treatment, also viewed the child's behavior as something that was bad.

A second component of this attitude about hyperactive children is that this behavioral disorder reflects something wrong with
the child, probably a disorder of his organic functioning if not the
organic structure. The organ generally implicated in this guilt is
the brain, thus we find an easy interchange among such words as
hyperactive, hyperkinetic, minimal brain dysfunction and *minimal
brain damage.*

A third feature of this prevailing attitude is that it is necessary
to identify and describe the organic difficulty and give it a label
prior to instituting treatment. Since the thing that is wrong
is unknown and assumed to relate to how the body works, it is the
physician who is called upon to carry out much of the diagnostic

process or to participate in it. As a reflection of this, it is viewed as proper for professionals, including psychologists, to conduct multiple examinations in order to arrive at a diagnosis and to find out if the child really does have this condition known as *hyperactivity or hyperkinesis.*

A fourth aspect of this common attitude is that after we have established the diagnosis there will be available a treatment that we can give to the child, something that we can do to him that will make him better. The significant features of this anticipated treatment are that it will be administered outside the school, usually by a physician; that the treatment will be medical in nature, generally a drug; and that the supervision and evaluation of the treatment will be done in isolation from the school. It is expected that the help the child gets from this outside treatment will be reflected in improved behavior in the classroom. The popularity of this notion about a simple medical procedure as effective therapy for hyperactivity is reflected in the fact that between 150,000 and 300,000 children in the United States are taking drugs for management of hyperactivity (Bazell, 1971). Robin and Bosco (1973) found that two thirds of the teachers that they interviewed had had at least one child in their class at some time who was taking Ritalin. Since only 15 percent of those teachers had been asked by physicians for information about how the child was getting along in school, it suggests that the bulk of children on drugs are receiving a treatment program that is divorced from the classroom.

Another feature of this general attitude is the expectation that it is up to the parents to see that the child gets to the doctor with the information from the school about the child's problem behaviors and to follow through with his prescription.

There are two messages conveyed by this attitude. One is that whatever we choose to do in terms of labeling and management, we should keep it simple. From both school and parents the message is *Find out what is wrong, label it, and give the child something that will help clear up the problem.* A second implication of this attitude is that no one is really responsible for the treatment and outcome. The school's responsibility ends after identifying the problem and making the referral to the physician. The family's responsibility ends with taking the child to the physician to get a prescription. The physician's responsibility is to rule out organic disease and to write a prescription for something to manage the child's behavior. The child is not assigned any responsibility for his own behavior or for what happens to him. The subsequent effect is that, if the prescribed treatment does not work, no one is responsible for the failure of the program.

AN ALTERNATIVE VIEW OF HYPERACTIVITY

An adequate program of medical management for hyperactive children stems from conceptions about these children, their behavior and their environments that are at variance with the notions expressed in the attitude above.

First, a thorough program of management is based on the knowledge that the problem of a child referred because of hyperactivity is almost always a complex one which does not lend itself to a treatment plan based on the keep-it-simple strategy. The behavior problem is almost never characterized simply by excessive motor behavior expressed in socially inappropriate ways. Rather, these children, who are supposedly plagued only by high rates of activity, exhibit a range of disordered behavior. The effects of the child's behavior on his educational and family environments are pervasive. For each child there are generally multiple factors contributing to the development and to the maintenance of the problem; these associated variables will influence the way in which the child responds to treatment. Many of the auxiliary achievement and behavioral disorders have long-lasting effects. And, further, we do not yet have the knowledge to predict from either the observable behavior or the results of examinations which specific treatment or combination of treatments will be best for a given child.

Second, it is vital that the child's behavior be assessed in all of the environments in which it is a problem. Discovering the variety of settings in which the problem is expressed is one of the things that we must determine. The appropriate subject of the evaluation is the child's behavior and the functionally related environmental variables, not his central nervous system.

Third, an adequate program of treatment for hyperactive children places the responsibility for management with a team of people including the physician, relevant school personnel, the parents, and the child. Each member's responsibilities are spelled out ahead of time, preferably in terms of contractual objectives for each team member.

The medical management program detailed in this chapter is based upon these convictions about hyperactivity and its treatment, namely, the complexity of the disorder, the need to study it directly where it is occurring, and the importance of shared responsibility in its management.

THE PREPARATORY EVALUATION

Developmental History of the Child

We begin the management program with an initial work-up that has several steps. The evaluation begins with a complete developmental history of the child taken from the parents, the purpose of which is to look at his patterns of physical growth, his motor development, speech and language development, and history of significant illnesses. Through this history we learn of factors that may have set the stage for the development of the behavior that is later labeled hyperactivity. A detailed history is also important in learning about the role of the child's behavior in the way that his family responds to him. Through the history we are essentially trying to identify any of the many things that could have interfered with normal progress through the developmental stages in which the child grows in size, strength and skill, in which he explores his world, and learns techniques of both social interaction and personal independence.

A compromising neonatal history or a lengthy illness in infancy may lead to parental expectations that the child will be abnormal, thus any deviant behavior is accepted as a fulfillment of this expectation. Inadequate parental information about normal toddler behavior may lead to labeling of legitimate exploratory behavior when the child is learning to walk as bad or abnormal. If this is combined with inappropriate child management techniques on the part of the parents, the behavior which is appropriate for very young children may be maintained through later periods while continuing to be viewed as abnormal. It is also important to know if there exists a parenting style that restricts exploratory behavior or prohibits autonomous decision making by the child since these restrictions frequently serve only to prevent the child from learning appropriate ways of acting independently.

The information gained from a complete developmental history will not predict what therapy is going to be the most effective, but it is an important step in the management plan since it aids in understanding the parents' reactions to the child's disorder and provides clues about how they can be expected to function in the treatment regime. The value of a detailed behavioral history in managing the hyperactive child has been pointed out by Wender (1971) and Bax (1971), who feel that a careful history may supply sufficient information to eliminate the need for other elaborate studies of the child. Understanding the development of the disorder is also useful in the broad task of prediction and prevention of child behavior disorders.

Examination of the Child

During the initial work-up it is important to obtain a complete picture of the child's physical status. The goal of the evaluation is not to establish a diagnosis or to seek that *thing that he has wrong,* but to understand completely his health status and to rule out those many conditions which masquerade as a behavioral disorder. For example, allergies represent the most common chronic health problem of childhood, affecting 14 percent to 24 percent of children (Kantor, 1974), and frequently they are not recognized. Yet, complaints of restlessness, disturbed sleep and increased motor activity are common in children with allergic reactions (Kittler, 1974), the same behaviors which characterize the hyperactive child. The Allergic-Tension-Fatigue syndrome (Speer, 1958) includes children described as hyperactive. A child with an unrecognized high-frequency hearing loss is another type of child who often presents himself with a pattern of behavior which is readily labeled as hyperactive. Behavioral disorders are frequent attendants to problems related to inadequate parenting such as poor nutrition and rest, or improper medical care and follow-through for chronic health problems such as parasitic disease, urinary tract infection and abdominal pain. We propose that any child who is referred to a physician with complaints of hyperactivity is entitled to the same complete pediatric study as any other child, which he frequently fails to get.

Referring a child with a behavioral disorder to make certain that the above kind of pediatric evaluation has been done is not the same as the common practice of referring every child perceived as hyperactive for a neurological to see if he has brain damage. The specialized tools of neurology such as the EEG and the brain scan are useful when the physician feels he has reason to rule out a seizure disorder, a tumor or a degenerative brain disease. It has been pointed out by reputable researchers and practitioners in the treatment of hyperactivity that it is not necessary for a child with uncomplicated hyperactivity to see a neurologist for the diagnosis of hyperactivity and, further, that the information from the specialized neurological tools are among the least helpful in developing a plan of management for these children (Kenny et al., 1971; Werry, 1968a, 1968b; and Werry and Sprague, 1970). The neurological component of the examination of the child referred for problem behavior can be done adequately by any physician willing to take the time to do so. Yet nonmedical referring personnel often question the adequacy of the evaluation if the child has not been given a complete neurological work-up.

When the physical examination of the child reveals problems in addition to the reported hyperactivity, such as clumsiness or awkwardness or a delay in the development of coordinated perceptual motor functioning, we deal with these as potential problem areas and make referrals to other disciplines such as occupational or physical therapy to explore remediation of these problems. It is not necessary to go beyond these associated problems and infer an underlying neurological problem since these so-called soft signs do not necessarily indicate that such a problem is the major cause of his behavioral disability.

We must draw a clear distinction between findings that hyperactivity is a behavioral feature of some children with confirmed brain injury (Clements, 1966 and Denhoff, 1973) and the relevance of seeking organic signs in all children presenting themselves with a behavioral problem of hyperactivity. When we start with groups of hyperactive children we find reported only a slightly increased incidence of mild neurological signs (Satterfield et al., 1972 and Werry and Sprague, 1970) and no differences from matched groups of EEG abnormalities (Werry et al., 1972). Even the notion of hyperactivity as a necessary component of brain injury is not supported by all findings (Werry, 1968b and Werry and Sprague, 1970). At the present time the hypothesis of the organic etiology of hyperactivity is not only of questionable validity, but, more importantly, its relevance in dictating therapy choices or predicting treatment outcome is in doubt (Freeman, 1970 and Werry, 1968).

This distinction between findings of hyperactivity among brain injured children and the value of identifying neurological signs in children whose presenting complaint is hyperactivity was not clearly made by some of the early writers in the area of the management of such children. There were at least three kinds of constitutional explanations of hyperactivity in the literature with similar terms often having different referents. One point of view related hyperactivity to damage to the brain or at least to brain dysfunction (Clements, 1966 and Stewart, 1970) with the possibility that we were not yet adequately sophisticated in assessment to find the damage. Another point of view related hyperactivity to a problem of brain process (Solomons, 1965) which is again difficult to assess clinically. A third kind of constitutional explanation is that represented by the work of Cruickshank who justified the use of the term *brain injured* to descriptively encompass the hyperactive child even though there was admittedly no demonstrable lesion since these children usually functioned like children with lesions (Cruickshank, 1967). These confusing early diagnostic conceptions are partly responsible for the commonly held notion that adequate management of the hyperactive child must start with in-depth neurological studies and end with medical treatment.

Current Educational Functioning

Another important part of the initial work-up of the child is the collection of information about his academic and behavioral status in the classroom. We must know the course of his educational progress and how his current achievement compares to age expectancies and be assured that his educational programming is based on current psychoeducational assessments. This information should be collected routinely because of the high incidence of academic problems encountered in children with complaints of hyperactivity (Clements, 1966; Keogh, 1971; and Laufer and Denhoff, 1957). We must also know about his nonacademic classroom behaviors since much of the vicious cycle of behavior difficulties such as low self-esteem, discouragement, misbehavior and poor achievement is centered in the classroom (Arnold, 1973a). It is also important to know how the child is being responded to by his teacher in terms of how she programs for him and what types of management procedures she is using. We must also know this teacher's notions about hyperactivity. Arnold suggests that we find out how many children in her class she is labeling hyperactive and compare this incidence with base rate frequencies (Arnold, 1973b).

The information about the child's difficulties in the classroom must be in terms of the specific problem behaviors directly observed by a reliable informant rather than indirect teacher reports that a child is hyperactive. As Bax states "True hyperkinetic syndrome is a rare disorder, the child who is regarded as overactive is a common problem" (Bax, 1971). Direct observation of the child in the classroom is necessary because of the indiscriminant faulty labeling of children as hyperactive when they are engaging in other deviant behavior even though restlessness, excitability or distractibility are not part of their deviant behaviors. The rate of the child's problem behaviors need not be high, just higher than the tolerance level of the teacher.

The need for physicians working with these children to be thoroughly familiar with school information and the facilities available to the children is stressed by many who have worked extensively with the treatment of hyperactivity (Bax, 1971; Feighner and Feighner, 1974; and Werry, 1968b). Many physicians feel that the collection of this information is difficult because of their time limits or because when they ask schools for this kind of material all they get are psychological reports listing subtest scores on an intelligence test. A satisfactory way of handling this problem is to set up a cooperative team including the physician, school psychologist, teacher, nurse, nonprofessional specially trained observer, etc., which meets on a regular basis to discuss the children in the physician's practice. Data collected by this team, whether in the classroom or in the physician's office, can be pulled into focus at the regularly scheduled meetings where it can be updated when necessary.

At this point the preparatory work-up for the child referred from the school is complete. By this stage of the management program we have determined by direct contact with the school what the child is doing academically and behaviorally that leads to concern, we have explored the development of his disability with his parents and have begun to get an idea of how others have perceived and reacted to him. We have also formed a picture of his physical status and ruled out the possibility that his behavior disorders are being amplified, if not totally maintained, by a chronic health problem.

BASELINE OBSERVATION

The next step of the management program is often difficult for family and school personnel to comprehend. After we have identified the target problem behaviors we observe the child and collect information on the frequency and course of these behaviors for a minimum of two and as many as six weeks before treating the child. It is because this preliminary information is vital in determining treatment choice and evaluating outcome that close physical-school communication is important.

Collecting observational information on the child labeled *hyperactive* is important for a number of reasons. First is the problem of faulty labeling mentioned above. The term *hyperactive* is popularly assigned both to children who engage in low frequency of behavior that the adult judges to be highly unacceptable and to children who do a lot of undesirable things at a fairly high rate. The significant variable in the application of the label is not the absolute frequency of the behavior but that the problem(s) occurs more than the adult can accept. Among the children referred to our clinic not only labeled as hyperactive, but also being treated by medication for hyperactivity, were a boy whose primary behavior deviations consisted of climbing over the fence once or twice a day when called into the house and using the bushes or sidewalk rather than the toilet for elimination, and a five year old girl who left the table frequently at mealtimes at home (but not at snack time in preschool) and who had the embarrassing tendency to throw her arms around the legs of unfamiliar men in public. Other children so labeled include those children who are doing things common for their age group but whose parents lack information about normal child development or have no techniques for helping the child develop alternative behaviors easier for them to handle. A toddler expressing normal curiosity may run off in the grocery store or run out into the street, and if the parent has no idea of how to curb this, the child may be perceived and labeled as overactive. Also, a child receiving classroom materials that are too difficult and getting no assistance from the teacher will likely engage in off-task behaviors and again be labeled as overactive. Douglas reports that her students' classroom observations of children judged to be hyperactive revealed that these children engaged in a lot of purposive behavior but which was unrelated to the activity of the rest of the class; their behavior was not random, but their goals were different from the teacher's (Douglas, 1972).

Thus, we cannot rely solely on parent or teacher report that a child is hyperactive but must confirm the presence of a significant number of the following behaviors which are those agreed upon as the significant components of hyperactivity: (1) distractibility, (2) short attention span, (3) overactivity or increased body movements, (4) restlessness such as finger tapping or fiddling, (5) excitability, (6) unpredictable mood changes, (7) explosive outbursts of anger or exasperation, (8) rapid changes in goal direction, (9) poor memory and (10) aggressiveness in peer relationships.

Baseline information from the classroom is also important because the problem may be environmentally specific such that something that occurs with alarming frequency in the classroom cannot be studied in other settings. Kenny and colleagues described the characteristics of one hundred children referred to their interdisciplinary clinic team because of hyperactivity. In only 25 percent of a total of 299 staff observations was a child judged to be overly active. The majority of the children were not considered hyperactive by any of the staff, and only thirteen of the one hundred were judged to be hyperactive by all professional observers. The lack of agreement about hyperactivity between classroom and clinic was particularly true of the children who were over age eight when referred and who had not been seen as unusually active until after age five (Kenny et al., 1971).

The baseline observation period allows teachers and parents to decide on the pinpoint priorities, which can be a difficult task for a number of reasons. The hyperactive child generally exhibits a broad repertoire of problem behavior. Stewart (1970) lists twenty-seven different parent complaints occurring in over 40 percent of his sample of hyperactive children. The initial presenting complaint may have been distorted as a result of teacher or parent reporting after an extreme day; this distortion is one reason for avoiding single observation assessment of these children. Extended observation also allows us to visualize the amount of day-to-day variability in the child's behavior.

Another reason for the observation period is that the problem behavior may fade with recording; the modifying effect of observation and recording alone is a well known phenomenon in the field of application of direct behavioral measurement; thus, this initial period is not really a baseline condition since by this time we have introduced several significant variables. The teacher knows that something is being done about the child's problem and this may affect her responses to him; the child knows that something is being done about him and this can easily alter his behavior. The modifying effect of observation alone dictates the need for good pretreatment information so that when we institute treatment we know that we are measuring treatment effects and not recording effects.

The major value of the observation period is that it allows us to identify some of the complicating child and environmental variables that are significant in the maintenance of the problem and will affect treatment. It is at this point that we recognize the parent who cannot remember appointments or reliably report on the child's behavior or the teacher who protests to her administrator her inclusion in the treatment program when she only wanted the child removed from her class. Not only can we assess the potential cooperation of parents and school personnel at this time, but we begin to get an idea of the other problems that will need to be dealt with. The hyperactive child is seldom one who is normal in all respects except for a high rate of motor activity; his hyperactivity is embedded in a complex social and behavioral system. Werry (1968b) fittingly refers to him as a multihandicapped child. These children encounter serious difficulties in the academic setting. Douglas, summarizing the characteristics of the children seen over a period of years at McGill University, reports that 70 percent of the hyperactive children had failed a grade by the time they were twelve and their grades were significantly lower than controls in almost all subjects (Douglas, 1972). Keogh (1971) points out several ways that hyperactivity may interact with learning to the detriment of the child's achievement. Freibergs and Douglas' findings that hyperactive children could do as well as normals on a concept learning task under continuous reinforcement, but did much worse than normals under partial reinforcement indicates that their learning difficulties reflect an interaction of attention and information variables and the way in which they receive consequences (Freibergs and Douglas, 1969).

Other complicating variables arise from the frequent family problems among children referred for hyperactivity. Mendelson, Johnson and Stewart (1971) report a higher incidence of drinking problems among the parents and a history of learning or behavior problems in parents or siblings. Other studies have also reported a higher incidence of psychiatric diagnoses in both parents and alcoholism among the fathers of hyperactive children (Cantwell, 1972 and Morrison and Stewart, 1971). Barcai (1969) also points out how parents' neurotic disorders can play a role in the maintenance of a child's hyperactivity.

Our awareness of the existence of these child, family and classroom variables before we institute treatment will increase the sophistication of our management program. It will keep us from prescribing a treatment that is unrealistic for parents to carry out, help us spot problem areas before they disrupt treatment, and help us sort out reasons for the changes in behavior during the management program.

The behavioral observations collected on the child in the classroom should ideally be made daily. One observation tactic is to obtain daily frequency counts of the target behaviors which have been pinpointed as the most prominent components of the child's disorder. Another option which is currently being used in a longitudinal controlled study of drug effects conducted by the second author is a direct observation technique adapted by Nelson (1971) from one developed by Werry and Quay (1969). In this technique the child is observed for two 20-second periods each minute for a fifteen-minute block of time, and his behavior is checked in terms of its classification into on or off task, deviant or teacher-child interaction categories. In the drug study we are collecting target data on the children sitting on all four sides of the subject in the classroom so that his behavior can be assessed against that of his peers. The value of direct behavioral observation in the evaluation of the hyperactive child has been demonstrated in the classroom (Becker, et al., 1967; Patterson, et al., 1965; and Werry and Quay, 1969) and in the laboratory (Doubros and Daniels, 1966). It reduces raters' bias so prevalent in many of the drug studies in that the parents and teachers who have a vested interest in the child rate the extent of his behavior change. The observation method selected should be determined partly by the availability of observers. If the teacher is to be the recorder, the number of behaviors studied may be fewer than if we have a trained observer who can spend time each day in the classroom. But direct, continuous observation of problem behavior children is so important to their management that a nonprofessional trained observer should be considered a vital member of the team.

SELECTION OF TREATMENT OPTIONS
The Planning Conference

Following the observation period of at least two weeks the physician, the family, the child and someone from the school meet to discuss the treatment options. The purpose of this meeting is to assure that each person is aware of the treatment selected and is involved in the decision, and to set up a management program that fosters open communication among all members of the participating team. There are a number of treatment tactics that are appropriately considered, and seldom is a single treatment sufficient. In a careful program the treatments are chosen on the basis of an analysis of the child's problems and the significant variables in the settings in which the behaviors occur.

Educational Intervention

One management tactic centers around changes in the child's educational environment. It is not unusual that a child with inappropriate classroom behavior is one receiving inadequate programming. Educational assessment and planning is not within the physician's province, but his responsibility includes knowing about the adequacy of the child's education, which means that direct communication with the school is mandatory. Interventions to consider may range from changes in the way in which curricular materials are programmed, changing teachers or transfer to a different type of classroom.

Direct Modification of Hyperactive Behavior

Another treatment tactic is the direct modification of hyperactivity in the significant environment by the systematic use of behavior management techniques. The decision for the team is really whether the behavior management program will be the only treatment undertaken or whether it will be used with additional

therapies since all of the components of this approach are important in dealing with hyperactive children. These elements are, first,
direct and continuous measurement of the problem behaviors in
their natural environment; second, relating their occurrence to
events in the environment which are discovered to be functionally
related; and, third, directly changing the frequency of the problem
behaviors by altering their relationships to these environmental
events, generally doing so by instructing parents and teachers in
techniques of behavior management. The value of this approach
as the sole treatment for hyperactive children has been clearly
demonstrated. Patterson and his colleagues were among the first to
report the modification of hyperactivity in the classroom by the
application of a set of contingent events designed to change the
frequency of the motor and speech activities that comprised the
disorder (Patterson et al., 1965). Twardosz and Sajwaj (1972)
found that a direct management program not only altered the
motor behavior of a hyperactive retarded child but had beneficial
effects on other play behaviors as well. Doubros and Daniels
(1966), using a contingent application of tokens for play and the
absence of hyperactive behaviors, reduced hyperactivity among
mentally retarded boys in a playroom setting. Daniels (1973) used
contingent parental attention to reduce hyperactivity in a child
with an additional physical disorder.

Drug therapy combined with behavior modification has been
suggested as a potent treatment tool. Werry and Sprague (1970)
describe the way in which the two treatments can work together.
They view drugs as aiding the behavior management program in
some cases by reducing the frequency of the hyperactive motor behaviors, but they recommend behavior management as the primary treatment. They list the strengths of the latter approach as a
focus on what the child is doing, which is understandable to parents and teachers and ensures greater cooperation from them; the
fact that the techniques can be carried out by those in the environment rather than by scarce therapists; and, also, that because of
the origins in experimental psychology, this approach emphasized
the evaluation of treatment effects.

Placement Outside of the Home

Another treatment option is to move the child to an entirely different living environment. This should be given consideration when the child's problems cannot be managed totally within the classroom and when his parents at the present time are not able to manage him, to administer the necessary treatments or to cooperate with or learn from any training program. This option is occasionally necessary because of the significant amount of pathology found in families of children with hyperactivity. It is not uncommon that the child's behavioral disorder is merely the focus of an entire constellation of family disorganization. In many cases treatment of the child outside the home allows the family to work on the other problems so that the child can later return to a home which can provide him with a better environment.

Drug Treatment

Misconceptions

The use of psychotropic drugs for the management of hyperactivity is another option to consider. This is the treatment of choice for those who take the keep-it-simple approach to treatment. Drugs are erroneously viewed by many as quick and easy to use, requiring no extensive involvement on the part of anyone. Before discussing the appropriate management of a drug regime it is necessary to address some of the misconceptions about their effectiveness in altering behavior and their supposed simplicity.

The use of medication alone or as the primary treatment, although a common practice, is not warranted on the basis of what we have learned about the complexity of the problems of hyperactivity. The activity level of the child, which is the justification for the drug, is seldom the child's only problem. By the time the child is referred from the school for treatment he not only emits high rates of motor activity but also engages in disruptive behavior in the classroom, is behind academically, has problems getting along with other children, and is most likely being responded to by adults in inappropriate or at least ineffectual ways. Thus, his problem includes not only his own learned responses but the reactions of others to him. Drugs alone cannot be expected to make a significant impact on all of these facets of the problem. Also, it has been our experience that families can more easily avoid facing the additional problems that they and the child are having when drugs are prescribed as the primary treatment.

A second misconception about medication for hyperactive children is that there are available drugs with a predictable and positive influence on academic performance. The hope that the drug will make the child more open to learning is expressed in many of the referrals to physicians from schools. Many writers express the notion that stimulant medication will indirectly aid the child's learning problems since the drug can affect some of the significant behavioral parameters of school functioning. Conners and Rothschild (1968) relate the value of stimulants in facilitating learning to their ability to reduce impulsiveness and restlessness which lead to hasty responding and errors as well as to the drug's ability to increase general alertness. Keogh (1971) states that drugs may indirectly facilitate academic improvement by their ability to alter behavior in a more socially compatible direction and by changing activity level and attention. Others refer to the facilitating effects of drugs via their ability to improve concentration (Weiss, Minde, Douglas, Werry and Sykes, 1971) and sustained attention (Sykes, Douglas and Morgenstern, 1972).

In reality, there is no consistent body of evidence to either support or negate the value of drugs in assisting classroom learning. Freeman (1966) reviewed thirty years of research on effects of drugs on learning. He found that most studies, although referring to learning, were primarily concerned with use of stimulants to control disruptive behavior. He also found that problems of methodology were so significant as to override the evidence of drug effects. The dearth of evidence of the effects of medication on academic performance continues to this time.

A major tactic for studying drug effects on cognitive behavior has been to use pre- and postscores on intelligence tests of groups of children on medication for a period of a few weeks or months. These studies do not show consistent improvement in test scores attributable to drugs. Some report increases on various WISC scores (Greenberg, Deem and McMahon, 1972 and Knights and Hinton, 1969). Other studies report no medication effects on the same measures (Conners and Rothschild, 1968; Conrad, Dworkin, Shai and Tobiessen, 1971; and Weiss, Werry, Minde, Douglas and Sykes, 1968). Conrad et al. (1971) measured the effects of dextro-amphetamine on thirty-four test variables including test scores, motor activity and general behavior. He found significant drug effects on only eight of these variables, with medication showing greater effects on motor activity, and no effects on WISC scores or on reading or arithmetic as measured by the Wide Range Achievement Test. Weiss, Minde and Douglas et al. (1971) found "unpredictable but positive" effects of stimulants on some subtests of the WISC and ITPA.

A second approach to studying effects of drugs on cognitive behavior has investigated children's performance on laboratory tasks of learning. Again the findings do not consistently point to ways in which medication can predictably affect the child's ability to learn. Baxley (1973) found no effects of stimulant drugs on either recall of a series of instructions or digits or on a complex recall task. Freibergs, Douglas and Weiss (1968) found no systematic effects of a tranquilizer on a concept learning task. Other studies report positive effects of stimulant medication on laboratory tasks. Sprague, Barnes and Werry (1970) found that a stimulant increased correct responding and decreased reaction time in a two-choice discrimination learning task. Others report that stimulants, acting on sustained attention, enhance laboratory task performance (Cohen, Douglas and Morgenstern, 1971 and Sykes, Douglas and Morgenstern, 1972). Although the laboratory studies do demonstrate facilitating effects of stimulants, the findings have only minimal application at this time to the understanding of how drugs might aid classroom learning.

It is very seldom that investigators study drug effects on learning in hyperactive children by directly measuring classroom academic performance. Sulzbacher (1972) has published one of the few studies employing this tactic. He measured academic target behavior in three children, studying effects of Ritalin on correct and error responses in math, oral reading and reading workbook performance. The children's responses were highly individual; one child's math performance doubled with no corresponding increase in errors under Ritalin, while his language arts performance was lower under certain drug dosages; a second child's error rates in math increased under Ritalin while his writing improved; the third child showed no language arts effect and his error rates decreased under medication. Similar findings were reported by Barrish (1974) who studied the effects of Ritalin on academic behavior in six children. She found that Ritalin affected several types of behavior including percent correct on academic tasks, number of problems completed and percent of assignments finished; however, as in Sulzbacher's study, the drug effects were different in terms of magnitude of effect and type of behavior affected in the individual children.

Thus, the expectation that we will be able to modify the hyperactive child's learning difficulties by the use of medication is not based on complete information about the effects of stimulants on learning. There is no consistent body of information supporting the use of medication to aid learning and, likewise, there is no evidence that stimulant medication will impair the child's ability to learn. The few studies which have directly measured academic performance suggest that drug effects on hyperactive children's learning are highly individual.

A third aspect of medication which is not appreciated is that the rationale for its use or for the selection of one drug over another is not based on research adequate to make sound conclusions about its benefits. There are certain minimal requirements of a study of behavioral effects of drugs. De Long (1972) lists the following necessary components: (1) placebo control, (2) random assignment of subjects to placebo and drug conditions, (3) triple blind procedures, (4) uniform groups of subjects of sufficient size to permit statistical analysis, (5) detailed description and measurement of the children studied, (6) precise description of the measurements and the criteria by which they are to be evaluated, and (7) detailed description of the children's social setting. Sprague and Werry (1971) list additional requirements: (1) drugs administered in standard dosages with the full dosage range explored, (2) assurances that the child takes the drug, (3) standardized evaluations that have been used before and whose reliability and validity are known.

Much of the research on drugs for hyperactive children has suffered from several major inadequacies. Conclusions about effects in individual children are based on averaged results from groups of children with poor description of how the data was analysed; research on a limited sample of important behaviors; use of tests and frequently homemade rating scales of questionable reliability and validity; poor control of drug administration and dosages; and no attempt to deal with the multiple environmental variables functional in each case.

In one of the most important reviews of the literature on psychotropic medication for children Sulzbacher (1973) looked at 756 studies of drug effects. He found that 72.5 percent lacked even the minimal controls listed above, and only 3.8 percent used direct behavioral observation of the children being treated, although direct behavioral recording of individual subjects is a highly sensitive measure of drug effects in children (Hollis and St. Omer, 1972 and Sulzbacher, 1972). He also found that the significance of the drug effects reported by the authors was related to the rigor of the measures used. In those studies relying on the opinion of observers about improvement with medication, the number of studies finding significant drug effects was higher than those finding no drug effects; in studies using rating scales to assess improvement, the number of studies finding significant drug effects was equal to the number finding no drug effects; in studies using psychological test scores or direct behavioral measures, the number of studies demonstrating significant drug effects was less than those demonstrating no effects.

A fourth aspect of medication not generally understood is that there is very little rationale for the use of one stimulant drug rather than another, nor is there a predictable relationship between the child's behavior, diagnostic category or neurological findings and his response to medication. Some studies report that children with a greater number of soft neurological signs respond better to medication than other hyperactive children (Conrad and Insel, 1967 and Satterfield et al., 1973) but this finding is not supported by a consensus of studies. Weiss, Minde and Douglas et al. (1971) found no relationship between effects of stimulant drugs and EEG findings, neurological history or severity of hyperactivity. Freeman (1970) concluded from his extensive literature review that the diagnosis of minimal brain damage as a valid predictor of drug response was too loose a diagnostic conception to use as a basis for prediction. Sprague and Werry (1971) conclude that the only way to predict whether a child will respond in the desired direction to drugs is to observe his behavior both on and off the medication. The inability to predict drug responses was also the conclusion of a conference sponsored by the Department of Health, Education and Welfare (Office Child Devel., 1971). The individual subject studies of Barrish (1973) and Sulzbacher (1972) reported above also suggest that we cannot with assurance predict which behavioral components of the problem will be affected by medication in individual children.

One significant factor in our inability to predict with accuracy an individual child's drug response is because some of the most significant variables in behavior change may be factors other than medication. Sulzbacher (1973) reports studies in which observers' ratings were more influenced by their knowledge of when crossover from drug to placebo occurred than by the actual medication change. The power of the placebo effect in children's response to medication is another of these powerful variables (Arnold, 1973 and McDermott, 1965).

Value of Drugs

Rather than the sole treatment tactic for hyperactivity medication is more appropriately considered an adjunct to a total management program. Werry and Sprague (1970) suggest its use to facilitate the emission of appropriate behavior in class such as sitting still and attending, which can then be strengthened by reinforcement procedures. The effects of medication have no permanence except as they indirectly lead to changes in the way that people in the child's environment respond to his behavior change (Werry, 1968b). The importance of viewing stimulants as only one component of the treatment program is stressed by many who have had extensive experimental and clinical experience with these children (Conners, 1973 and Werry, 1968b).

Although both tranquilizers and stimulants are prescribed for hyperactive children, the latter (either methylphenidate [Ritalin] or dextroamphetamine [Dexedrine®]), are preferred because they have fewer side effects and have demonstrated equal if not more positive effects on behavior (Weiss, Minde, Douglas et al., 1971 and Werry, 1970). The main effect of the stimulants, based on a consensus of field studies, has been a reduction of disruptive motor activity in some of the children treated. The main process effects of the medication based on behavioral studies in the laboratory are interpreted as the facilitation of sustained attention and a reduction of impulsive response to tasks (Douglas, 1972 and Werry, 1970).

The Drug Treatment Regime

A medical management program for hyperactivity that uses drugs in a valid way requires that a number of contingencies be set up. Much of the rationale for these contingencies has been presented above and will only be referred to summarily here.

1. The physician must have access to the important people in the child's environment. This includes the parents and school personnel as well as the child himself. The hyperactive child's problems, as stressed in this chapter, are generally many faceted; they are troublesome to teachers and parents and cannot be dealt with in isolation from these adults.

2. Baseline observations of the child in his important settings must be collected consistently over a long enough period of time, generally two to six weeks, to allow for initial observation effects to occur and to gain an adequate picture of what the child is doing.

3. After the child is on medication the behavioral observation and data collection must continue in the classroom. There must be

provision for immediate assessment of any significant behavior change that may occur, which is only possible when school and medical personnel are available to each other.

4. Parents and school personnel must have, in writing, complete information about the prescription and should sign contracts that the medication will be given as prescribed, in the prescribed dosage, and that it will not be stopped or altered without consulting the physician.

5. When the initial therapy planning conference is held it is important that part of the contract be set up with the child. He should be completely informed about the medication regime and take as much responsibility as possible for his own medication.

6. The child must be seen by the physician on a regular basis. The schedule varies with individual children from once a week to once every three to four weeks. When the child is on medication it is important that the physician monitor his growth and general health, including appetite, blood pressure and pulse ratings, and explore any complaints indicating side effects of the medication.

7. The decision needs to be clearly established at the start of treatment whether the medication is to be given on a trial basis with behavioral data collected to determine its appropriateness for the child or if it is to be used with other treatment procedures such as a classroom change or a behavioral management program. In a careful drug program it is important that the introduction of alternate treatment is done in an orderly manner and is carefully documented. If medication is used with other procedures it is wise to use control periods during which the effects of each can be assessed.

Contraindications

Medication for hyperactivity is not indicated for children under age five and for those who have multiple complex medical problems in which case alternative treatment programs must be outlined. Medication is contraindicated or is terminated if there are any environmental variables which will make it difficult for the child to take the medication as prescribed or if any problems such as lack of family responsibility for the treatment plan, lack of school cooperation or limited recording of the child's behavior will preclude the necessary contingencies from being met. It has been our experience that in many cases, rather than relying on these criteria, drugs are prescribed for just the opposite reasons—when there is no way of working directly with the family, when the problems associated with the child's behavior are so complex that it is difficult to sort out the interrelations of problem behaviors and sustaining events, and when there is only limited access to the child or to the school. Drugs should not be continued over a period of a few years without a monitoring system for what is happening to the child's behavior and to his environment. In order to evaluate the child's behavior and the direction and extent of change it is vital that the objectives for the treatment program and thus the criteria for evaluating it be set up at the time of the initial treatment planning conference.

FOLLOW THROUGH

Whatever the treatment options, a comprehensive program continues with periodic conferences of the relevant people which have been scheduled ahead of time. Regular meetings for review of the child's behavioral and academic records and medical status allow us to keep current about treatment effects, whether of drugs or other programs. These meetings are an efficient way for all who are working with the child to update their information about what is happening in all settings.

Continuous monitoring of the behavior while treatments are in effect is necessary to free our assessment of the child's progress from the frequent mismatch between the child's behavior change and reports about that change. Despite evidence for this discrepancy, the bulk of drug research has relied on parent or teacher reports about children's previous behavior changes, and this continues to be the way most clinical cases are evaluated. By monitoring the child continuously the treatment team can also more easily identify, measure the effects of, and deal with the potent extra treatment variables that influence the child's behavior, perhaps even more than the treatment we have prescribed. These variables may include changes in school personnel or curriculum or events that influence the parents' behavior. It is only when we can relate the child's behavior change to these environmental events at the time that they are happening that we can clearly analyse their effects.

SUMMARY

The management program outlined in this chapter is not the quick and easy one that the school and parents often expect will be prescribed, but one involving many facets that are vital to the management of the complex problem of hyperactivity.

The first component relates to the way in which we describe and assess the child's problem. This includes focusing on what the child does in significant environments and how he is responded to. It also includes ruling out medical or other behavioral problems which are mislabeled as hyperactivity rather than carrying out assessments to rule in this elusive condition.

The second component relates to the way we measure the severity of the disorder and the direction of behavior change. This component stresses direct and continuous behavioral measurement of important behaviors such as disruptive acts and academic performance in settings in which they occur over a sufficient period of time before and during treatment. This type of measurement is recommended as the best way to deal with problems of rater's bias inaccurate reporting of frequency and changes in problem behavior unrelated to our prescribed treatment.

The third component relates to our analysis of the multiple variables that influence the child's behavior and how we seek to identify them and use them to the child's benefit rather than prescribe a simple or single treatment which may be less powerful than these environmental variables.

We feel that all of these components of a treatment program are important in the management of the hyperactive child, and these require a longitudinal program. It is thus apparent that adequate medical management is not something that occurs just by going to the physicians' office but is a broader spectrum of evaluation and treatment using a team of people who are willing to participate in the program by assisting in collection of data that will help us define the child's problem, assure that the treatment program is being administered, and participate in the updating of information about the direction of the child's behavior change.

REFERENCES

Arnold, L. E.: Is this label necessary? *J Sch Health,* 43(8):510-514, 1973.
Arnold, L. E.: The art of medicating hyperkinetic children. *Clin Pediatr,* 12(1):35-41, 1973.
Barcai, A.: The emergence of neurotic conflict in some children after successful administration of dextroamphetamine. *J Child Psychol Psychiatry, 10:*269-276, 1969.
Barrish, H. H.: Ritalin as the independent variable in a reversal design. Unpublished doctoral dissertation, University of Kansas, 1973.
Bax, M.: The larger half. *Dev Med Child Neurol, 13:*135-136, 1971.
Baxley, J. B.: Effects of psychotropic drugs on the short-term memory of retarded children. Unpublished doctoral dissertation, University of Kansas, 1973.
Bazell, R. J.: Panel sanctions amphetamines for hyperkinetic children. *Science, 171:*1223, 1971.
Becker, W. C., Madsen, C. H., Arnold, C. R., and Thomas, D. R.: The contingent use of teacher attention and praise in reducing classroom behavior problems. *J Spec Ed, 1:*287-307, 1967.
Cantwell, D. P.: Psychiatric illness in the families of hyperactive children. *Arch Gen Psychiatry, 27(3):*414-417, 1972.
Clements, S. D.: Minimal Brain Dysfunction in Children. (NINDB Monograph No. 3, U.S. Public Health Service Publication). Washington, D.C., U.S. Government Printing Office, 1966.
Cohen, N. J., Douglas, V. I., and Morgenstern, G. G.: The effect of methylphenidate on attentive behavior and autonomic activity in hyperactive children. *Psychopharmacologia, 22:*282-294, 1971.
Conners, C. K.: What parents need to know about drugs and special education. *J Learning Disabil, 6(6):*349-355, 1973.
Conners, C. K., and Rothschild, G. H.: Drugs and learning in children. In Hellmuth, J. (Ed.): *Learning Disorders.* Seattle, Special Child, 1968, vol. 3.
Conrad, W. G., Dworkin, E. S., Shai, A., and Tobiessen, J. E.: Effects of amphetamine therapy and prescriptive tutoring on the behavior and achievement of lower class hyperactive children. *J Learn Disabil,* 4(9): 509-517, 1971.
Conrad, W. G., and Insel, J.: Anticipating the response to amphetamine therapy in the treatment of hyperkinetic children. *Pediatrics, 40:*96-98, 1967.

Cruickshank, W. M.: *The Brain Injured Child in Home, School, and Community.* Syracuse, Syracuse U Pr, 1967.

Daniels, L. K.: Parental treatment of hyperactivity in a child with ulcerative colitis. *J Beh Ther Exp Psychiatry, 4*:183-185, 1973.

De Long, R.: What have we learned from psychoactive drug research on hyperactives? *Am J Dis Child, 123*:177-180, 1972.

Denhoff, E.: The natural life history of children with minimal brain dysfunction. *Ann NY Acad Sci, 205*:188-205, 1973.

Doubros, S. G., and Daniels, G. J.: An experimental approach to the reduction of overactive behavior. *Beh Res Ther, 4*:251-258, 1966.

Douglas, V. I.: Stop, look and listen: The problem of sustained attention and impulse control in hyperactive and normal children. *Can J Behav Sci, 4*(4):259-282, 1972.

Feighner, A. C., and Feighner, J. P.: Multi-modality treatment of the hyperkinetic child. *Am J Psychiatry, 131*(4):459-463, 1974.

Freeman, R. D.: Drug effects on learning in children: A selective review of the past thirty years. *J Spec Ed, 1*(1):17-44, 1966.

Freeman, R. D.: Review of medicine in special educ.: Another look at drugs. *J. Spec Ed, 4*(3):377-384, 1970.

Freibergs, V., and Douglas, V. I.: Concept learning in hyperactive and normal children. *J Abnorm Psychol, 74*:388-395, 1969.

Freibergs, V., Douglas, V. I., and Weiss, G.: The effect of chlorpromazine on concept learning in hyperactive children under two conditions of reinforcement. *Psychopharmacologia, 13*:299-310, 1968.

Greenberg, L. M., Deem, M. A., and McMahon, S.: Effects of dextroamphetamine, chlorpromazine and hydroxyzine on behavior and performance in hyperactive children. *Am J Psychiatry, 129*(5):532-539, 1972.

Hollis, J. H., and St. Omer, V. V.: Direct measurement of psychopharmacologic response: Effects of chlorpromazine on motor behavior of retarded children. *Am J Ment Defic, 76*(4):397-407, 1972.

Kantor, J. M.: Incidence of allergy in childhood. In Speer, F., and Dockhorn, R. (Eds.): *Allergy and Immunology in Children.* Springfield, Thomas, 1973.

Kenny, T. J., Clemmens, R. L., Hudson, B. W., Lenz, G. A., Cicci, R., and Nair, P.: Characteristics of children referred because of hyperactivity. *J Pediatrics, 79*(4):618-622, 1971.

Keogh, B. K.: Hyperactivity and learning disorders: Review and speculation. *Except Child, 38*:101-107, 1971.

Kittler, F. J.: Allergy and behavior. In Speer, F., and Dockhorn, R. J. (Eds.): *Allergy and Immunology in Children.* Springfield, Thomas, 1973.

Knights, R. M., and Hinton, G. G.: The effects of methylphenidate (Ritalin) on the motor skills and behavior of children with learning problems. *J Nerv Ment Dis, 148*:643-53, 1969.

Laufer, M. W., and Denhoff, E.: Hyperkinetic behavior syndrome in children. *J Pediatrics, 50:*463-73, 1957.

McDermott, J. F.: A specific placebo effect encountered in the use of dexadrine in a hyperactive child. *Am J Psychiatry, 121:*923-24, 1965.

Mendelson, W., Johnson, N., and Steward, M.: Hyperactive children as teenagers: A follow-up study. *J Nerv Ment Dis, 153:*273-79, 1971.

Morrison, J. R., and Stewart, M. A.: A family study of the hyperactive child syndrome. *Biol Psychiatry, 3:*189-95, 1971.

Nelson, C. M.: Techniques for screening conduct disturbed children. *Except Child, 37:*501-8, 1971.

Office of Child Development, Department of Health, Education, and Welfare. Report on the conference on the use of stimulant drugs in the treatment of behaviorally disturbed young school children. *Psychopharmacol Bull, 7:*23-9, 1971.

Patterson, G. R., Jones, R., Whittier, J., and Wright, M. A.: A behavior modification technique for the hyperactive child. *Behav Res Ther, 2:* 217-26, 1965.

Robin, S. S., and Bosco, J. J.: Ritalin for school children: The teachers' perspective. *J Sch Health, 43*(10):624-28, 1973.

Satterfield, J. H., Cantwell, D. P., Lesser, L. I., and Podosin, R. L.: Physiological studies of the hyperkinetic child: I. *Am J Psychiatry, 128:*1425-1431, 1972.

Satterfield, J. H., Cantwell, D. P., Saul, R. E., Lesser, Li. I., and Podosin, R. L.: Response to stimulant drug treatment in hyperactive children: Prediction from EEG and neurological findings. *J Autism Child Schizo, 3*(1):36-48, 1973.

Solomons, G.: The hyperactive child. *J Iowa Med Soc, 15*(8):464-69, 1965.

Speer, F.: The allergic-tension-fatigue syndrome in children. *Int Arch Allergy, 12:*207-214, 1958.

Sprague, R .L., Barnes, K. R., and Werry, J. S.: Methylphenidate and thioridazine: Learning, reaction, time, activity, and classroom behavior in disturbed children. *Am J Orthopsychiatry, 40*(4):615-628, 1970.

Sprague, R. L., and Werry, J. S.: Methodology of psychopharmacological studies with the retarded. In Ellis, N. R. (Ed.): *International Review of Research in Mental Retardation.* New York, Acad Pr, 1971, vol. 5.

Stewart, M. A.: Hyperactive children. *Sci Am, 222*(4):94-98, 1970.

Sulzbacher, S. I.: Behavior analysis of drug effects in the classroom. In Semb, George (Ed.): *Behavior Analysis and Education,* University of Kansas, 1972.

Sulzbacher, S. I.: Psychotropic medication with children: An evaluation of procedural biases in results of reported studies. *Pediatrics, 51*(3):513-517, 1973.

Sykes, D. H., Douglas, V. I., and Morgenstern, G.: The effect of methylphenidate (Ritalin) on sustained attention in hyperactive children. *Psychopharmacologia, 25*(3):262-74, 1972.

Twardosz, S., and Sajwaj, T.: Multiple effects of a procedure to increase sitting in a hyperactive, retarded boy. *J Appl Beh Anal, 5*:73-78, 1972.

Weiss, G., Minde, K., Douglas, V., Werry, J., and Sykes, D.: Comparison of the effects of chlorpromazine, dextroamphetamine and methylphenidate on the behavior and intellectual functioning of hyperactive children. *Can Med Assoc J, 104*:20-5, 1971.

Weiss, G., Werry, J., Minde, K., Douglas, V., and Sykes, D.: Studies on the hyperactive child: V. The effects of dextroamphetamine and chlorpromazine on behavior and intellectual functioning. *J Child Psychol Psychiatry, 9*:145-156, 1968.

Wender, P. H.: *Minimal Brain Dysfunction in Children.* New York, Wiley, 1971.

Werry, J. S.: Developmental hyperactivity. *Pediatr Clin North Am, 15*(3): 581-99, 1968a.

Werry, J. S.: Some clinical and laboratory studies of psychotropic drugs in children: An overview. In Smith, W. L. (Ed.): *Drugs and Cerebral Function.* Springfield, Thomas, 1970.

Werry, J. S.: The diagnosis, etiology, and treatment of hyperactivity in children. In Hellmuth, J. (Ed.): *Learning Disorders.* Seattle, Special Child, 1968b, vol. 3.

Werry, J. S., Minde, K., Guzman, A., Weiss, G., Dogan, K., and Hoy, E.: Studies on the hyperactive child-VII: Neurological status compared with neurotic and normal children. *Am J Orthopsychiatry, 42*(3):441-450, 1972.

Werry, J. S., and Quay, H. C.: Observing the classroom behavior of elementary school children. *Except Child, 35*(6):461-67, 1969.

Werry, J. S., and Sprague, R. L. Hyperactivity. In Costello, C. G. (Ed.): *Symptoms of Psychopathology.* New York, Wiley, 1970.

3

A behavioral approach to the management of hyperactive behavior

Herbert J. Rieth

For over one hundred years, since its initial recognition by Hoffman (1844) as a separate and distinct behavioral characteristic, hyperactivity has been the subject of observation and formalized study. The extended length of study serves to highlight the concern regarding the management of hyperactivity. Patterson (1955) indicated that high rates of activity in the behavior of children are one of the most frequent complaints made by adults in referring children to outpatient clinics. Acting out and disruptive behaviors have been the behaviors most frequently selected by teachers as targets for projects completed as part of a classroom management course taught by the author. Cruickshank (1967) indicated that hyperactivity in all forms and degrees is one of the most significant hurdles to adjustment in home and in the school.

Given this concern, what can we as professionals offer to facilitate the management of hyperactivity? Obviously there are many theories and procedures proffered, and they vary in relevance and effectiveness. In this chapter one approach to the management of hyperactivity will be discussed and eight illustrative studies will be presented. The approach has been labeled a behavioral approach. The approach is not viewed as a panacea but as an effective tool in the practitioner's repertoire of skills to manage the behavior of hyperactive children.

DESCRIPTION OF A BEHAVIORAL APPROACH

What constitutes a "behavioral approach"? The behavioral approach focuses upon the behavior emitted by the person. Behavior as it will be used in this chapter was defined by Sulzer and Mayer (1972) as any observable external act of an organism. Consequently the behavioral approach to hyperactivity entails the observation and measurement of those behaviors emitted by the organism which can conceivably be categorized as falling under the rubric of hyperactivity. The approach is based upon the assumption that, regardless of their etiology, hyperactive behaviors can be controlled by the application of general principles of learning theory (Skinner, 1953 and Bijou and Baer, 1961). The practitioner employing the behavioral approach would be concerned with the behavior emitted by the organism and not with the etiology other than as it would be suggestive of a modification procedure for hyperactive behavior. This is an important distinction between this and other approaches.

Since the behavioral approach is relegated to the consideration of behaviors which are observable and measureable, it would appear important to attempt to relate hyperactivity to this paradigm. Keogh (1971), in commenting on the definition of hyperactivity, indicated that classroom teachers may well agree with the observation that "hyperactivity is like pornography, hard to define but you know it when you see it." In a related statement Keogh (1971) observed that part of the problem in research and program development has been the lack of the well-defined criteria needed to identify hyperactivity. In attempting to provide a criterion Werry, Minde, Guzman, Weiss, Dogan and Hoy (1972) defined hyperactivity as a chronic sustained level of motor activity which, because of its excessive degree, is the source of continued complaint from both the child's home and his other environments. This definition suggests that hyperactivity consists of a variety of behaviors and that complaints from the environment constitute the criterion for intervention. Schmitt et al. (1973) concurred and indicated that hyperactivity is not a diagnosis and not a syndrome; it is a behavior. The child is simply more active than the adults in his environment think he should be. Since hyperactivity is viewed as a behavior, one is confronted with the task of observing, measuring and modifying or changing this behavior.

Once a behavior is selected, the initial task becomes that of breaking it down into its component acts or operations. Thus, if a child is referred because he or she is hyperactive, then the practitioner employing the behavioral approach would work with the person making the referral to break hyperactive behavior down into its component parts. For example, one of the behaviors which frequently prompts the labeling of a child as hyperactive is *out-of-seat* behavior. In attempting to manage this behavior the first step is to designate what constitutes an out-of-seat. Generally, the behavior is defined as the child's buttocks leaving contact with the chair seat. With this definition the behavior can be reliably measured. In considering this example it should be mentioned that frequently it is necessary to differentiate authorized from unauthorized chair-leaving. The reason for the differentiation is that the students often don't know what the rule is regarding movement around the classroom, and the teacher doesn't know the reason for the out-of-seat unless she asks. The mere fact that the teacher poses the question of why the student is out of his seat may, in fact, maintain or increase out-of-seat behavior.

Another behavior which is frequently ascribed to hyperactivity is a *short attention span*. This term would obviously defy reliable measurement. This behavior could be broken down to attending to task, which has been defined by Rieth (1971) as looking at the appropriate assignment sheet or work materials. In addition, any contact with the teacher such as raising a hand for help or discussion of the assignment would constitute attending.

In group work, attending was described as orientation toward work materials, to a reciting fellow student, to the teacher or, if responding orally, to a lesson.

The definitions presented provide illustrations of how at least two of the behaviors associated with hyperactivity can be defined in terms that are observable and measureable. The true test of the accuracy of any definition, however, involves the collection of reliability data. Hall (1971) indicated that reliability checks are used to provide added confidence that it is indeed the behavior and not the observer's recording of the behavior which changes from one experimental condition to another. Reliability refers to the degree of agreement between independent observers making independent observations of the same behavior. Reliability is usually expressed in mathematical terms and can be calculated by dividing the number of agreements by the total number of observations and multiplying the quotient by 100. Hall (1971) indicated that there are no absolute standards that have been established, but generally 80 percent or better has been deemed acceptable for many behaviors.

Once a behavior is selected and defined, the next step in the process involves the measurement of the behavior. The mentioning of measurement usually prompts two statements. The first is "It isn't necessary to measure," and the second is "I don't have time to measure." The response to the first statement involves pointing out one of the primary reasons for measuring, which is to determine whether the procedure or treatment program is working. Thus, data in the form of repeated measures is necessary to determine if the level of the behavior is any different after treatment has been implemented than it was prior to the implementation of the treatment. The repeated measures necessitate, for the most part, recording a daily measure of the behavior which provides immediate feedback to the teacher or parent regarding the efficacy of the treatment program.

In response to the second statement, the feasibility of measuring is amply documented in the *Journal of Applied Behavior Analysis*, Hall, Vol. 3 (1971) and in the case studies at the end of the chapter. Behavior has been recorded by large numbers of people with few reports of measurement precluding the completion of other duties. The feasibility can be enhanced by the selection of the proper type of measurement. Hall (1971) listed three major types of measurement. They include automatic recording, direct measurement and observational recording. Since this presentation is relegated specifically to school and home settings, direct and certain types of observational recording will be discussed.

One type of measurement which is frequently employed is direct measurement of permanent products. This type of measurement can be used if one is interested in obtaining a measure of the written academic responses emitted by the child. Thus, if one is more interested in the academic rather than the social behavior or wishes to measure them concurrently, this would be a recommended type of measurement. This might be highly desirous since academic difficulties are frequently correlated with the occurrence of social behaviors that are labeled hyperactive. Keogh (1971) indicated that the question of why the child labeled as hyperactive has learning problems is not too clear. One hypothesis that might explain the academic difficulties is the fact that many of the social behaviors that have been responsible for the child being labeled hyperactive may be incompatible with the accurate completion of academic assignments. This would mean the fact that the child is out of his seat, roaming around the classroom, may be incompatible with the accurate completion of academic assignments.

One strategy which has been employed successfully has been to reinforce the child for emitting correct academic responses (see Case Study 3). The rationale for this strategy is that if the child is being reinforced for correct responses and the student is responding by sitting in his seat working on academics, this is incompatible with being out-of-seat, roaming around the classroom. This strategy assumes that the task is consonant with the student's academic repertoire. In the event that the task is not consonant, the task should be examined and a more appropriate task should be selected.

Cooper (1974) reported that teachers usually translate permanent products to numerical terms of (1) frequency of correct academic responses, (2) rate of correct academic responses, or (3) percentage of correct responses. Frequency of correct responses is typically used when the same number of responses is assigned or required during the data collection sessions. Rate of responses is defined as the frequency of academic response during a unit of time. Cooper (1974) indicated "that the relationship between correct and error rate generates the same type of information as is obtained with frequency and percentage measures." He added that, additionally, rate measures are sensitive to the proficiency of student performances since they are sensitive to the effects of teaching tactics on student responses because they will show very small increments of behavior change. A major drawback to this type of measurement, however, is the amount of teacher time necessary to monitor the rate measures. There are strategies available to reduce the amount of teacher involvement. One strategy which is often used involves training the students to record the time it takes them to complete an assignment.

The remaining type of measurement is observational recording. Hall (1971) listed six types of observational recording. They included continuous, event, duration, interval, time sample and placheck.

CONTINUOUS MEASUREMENT, as the name implies, involves recording behavior as it occurs. This type of measurement has only recently become available to the practitioner because of the development and increased accessibility, of media such as videotape or 8mm cameras to facilitate the recording of the diverse numerous behavioral episodes. The major disadvantage of this type of recording is that it would involve repeated monitoring to accurately record the data.

EVENT RECORDING is the most frequently used type of observational recording used to record hyperactivity. Hall (1971) indicated that in event recording an observer using event recording procedures makes a frequency count of discrete events of a certain class as they occur. Most of the hyperactive behaviors listed by Patterson (1966) would be measured using event recording. The behaviors listed included the inappropriate occurrence of talking, pushing, hitting, pinching, looking about the room, looking out the window, walking around the room, moving one's desk, tapping, squirming and handling objects. This type of recording is readily useable by most practitioners.

DURATION RECORDING. This method involves recording how long the person engages in the target behavior during the observation period. This type of recording is frequently used when the duration of a behavior is more reflective of the intensity of a behavior than the frequency of a behavior. This is exemplified by a student who doesn't leave his seat very often but when he leaves it he is out for a considerable period of time. In this case the durational recording would more accurately reflect the behavior than an event measurement.

INTERVAL RECORDING can be very effectively employed by observers other than the teacher or person responsible for monitoring classroom activities. This type of recording involves dividing the observation period into equal intervals. The observer then notes whether the target behavior occurs during a given interval. The behavior is expressed in the percent of occurrence. This type of measurement is frequently used to record attending behavior, which would make it useful in recording behaviors frequently grouped under hyperactivity.

TIME SAMPLING is similar to interval recording, however it does not require the continuous observation required by interval recording. This recording involves breaking the observation period up into equal intervals with the behavior being recorded only if it occurs at the end of each interval. Thus, this type of measurement can be employed easily by a teacher. An example of the utility of this type of measurement might involve the observation of attending behavior for a thirty-minute period with the behavior being observed and recorded every two minutes. Thus, every two minutes the teacher would look at the child and record whether or not he or she was paying attention.

PLACHECK (Planned Activity Check) was recently developed by Risley (1972). It is similar to time sampling in that the observation period is divided into equal intervals, and the behavior is observed at the end of the interval. This type is generally used for recording the behavior of a group of children and to measure how many are participating in the behavior or planned activity. If a teacher wanted to determine what portion of a preschool class is participating in language development activities, she would, at the end of each interval, record the number of students in the group who were participating. She would then divide that number by the number of children in the group and multiply the quotient by 100. This would yield the percent of participation. If, for example, there were ten students in the class and eight were participating, then 80 percent participation would be recorded. This would be done after each interval, and then a mean would represent the score for the entire observation period.

The preceding has provided a brief overview of the types of measurement that can be employed to obtain some idea of quantity of the behavior emitted by the child, or group, that the teacher wants changed. In addition, the data provides a numerical assessment of the effectiveness of the program devised to change the child's behavior.

Once the target behavior is selected and defined, measures are taken before treatment is implemented to determine the frequency or intensity of the behavior. These measures are called baseline measures and are taken until the behavior has attained a steady state (Sidman, 1960). This means that we can accurately predict the future level of the behavior if it is left untreated. Thus, we have a basis with which to compare the effect of the program devised to change the behavior. The criterion for the effectiveness of the intervention as stated by Baer, Wolf and Risley (1968) is that "if the application of behavioral techniques does not produce large enough effects for practical value then application has failed" and another procedure or technique should be applied.

MANAGEMENT TECHNIQUES

What are some of the techniques or procedures which can be employed to deal with behavior specifically, in this case hyperactivity? The procedures to be discussed will have the effects of increasing, maintaining or decreasing the postbaseline level of behavior. The management techniques to be discussed are reinforcement, extinction, punishment and antecedent events.

Reinforcement is defined as any event which follows a behavior which increases the probability that the behavior will occur in the future (Skinner, 1953). In many of the published studies the behaviors reinforced were incompatible with hyperactivity in order to increase the frequency of those behaviors and reduce the frequency of the hyperactivity. Patterson (1966) conducted a study with a child who was referred to a clinic because of marked hyperactive behavior and academic retardation. He was described as being in almost continuous motion in the classroom and impossible to control unless he was in the immediate presence of the teacher. Hyperactivity was described as the "inappropriate occurrence of the following behaviors: talking, pushing, hitting, pinching, looking about the room, looking out the window, moving out of location (walking or moving desk) and moving in location (clapping, squirming, handling object)." The frequency of each response was tabulated for each thirty-second interval during a twenty-minute observation period. A training procedure was initiated in a small cubicle in the clinic area when the child met individually with Patterson. The child sat at a table that had a device with a light bulb on top of it. The child was told that while he was in his seat the light bulb would be turned on in recognition of the fact that he was in his seat. Each time that it was turned on the child would earn either a piece of candy or a penny. Once the child was trained to respond appropriately, the apparatus was installed in the classroom. In this case the light was activated remotely by the experimenter who was sitting across the room. The other children were told of the intent of the program, then their cooperation was solicited and obtained. The main advantage of the light was that it facilitated the immediate presentation of the token reinforcer emitting the desired behavior. As a result of this procedure, along with the encouragement of his peers, the frequency of inappropriate behavior dropped from 16.0 to 4.6. It should be noted that initially the behavior was reinforced frequently; then, once established, the frequency of reinforcement was diminished. These are important points to monitor. The immediacy of reinforcement is very critical when one is attempting to build in a new behavior or increase the frequency of behavior.

The immediate presentation of the reinforcer clarifies the relationship between the reinforcer and the appropriate behavior. Another critical point is that the behavior should be reinforced frequently (continuously) when it is occurring at a low level in the youngster's behavioral repertoire.

Whitman, Coponigri and Mercurio (1971) employed tactics similar to Patterson (1966) when they reinforced behaviors which were incompatible with hyperactivity which in this case meant continuous movement around the classroom. The behaviors measured consisted of the latency in responding to the teacher's command to sit down, the number of commands to sit down, and the length of time the child spent sitting. When baseline was completed the authors instituted a training procedure which was first applied in a small room away from the classroom. Initially they began to reinforce the child for sitting down. If she was not in her seat attempts were made to get her attention and request that she sit down; if she complied she was reinforced. If she didn't respond she was guided to the chair by taking her hand and walking her to the chair. When she complied she was reinforced. If she did not comply she was then instructed to sit down, and if she did not respond she was guided into the chair. She was then reinforced for remaining in the chair. Reinforcers included praise, chocolate, raisins, cheese and crackers. Initially the student was reinforced for sitting in her seat for twenty seconds, and after she continually met criterion the sitting time required to earn the reinforcement was gradually increased. At the end of the training session the child was required to sit in her chair for two minutes in order to earn the reinforcer. When training was completed, generalization was assessed by placing her in the classroom and measuring her behavior. After training, over a twenty-minute observation period, the mean number of commands necessary to get her to sit was reduced from 17.8 to 2.8 while the latency between the issuance of the command and actual compliance was reduced 7.0 seconds. The amount of time she remained in her seat increased from 59.8 to 331.6 seconds. This occurred despite the fact that the teacher in no way reinforced the girl. The author speculated, however, that the statistics would have been even more impressive had the teacher implemented the reinforcement procedures which had proven so successful.

Examples of other reinforcers applied to different classes of behaviors can be found in the case studies at the end of this chapter. The reinforcers range from teacher praise and attention to token reinforcement procedures which had back-up reinforcers including small toys, trinkets, good worker, seat back covers, candy, animal stamps and soda pop. The variety of reinforcers used highlights the fact that different events serve as reinforcers for different people. Consequently, the practitioner must be ever vigilant to identify reinforcers for the child with whom they work. This task can, upon occasion, be expedited by observing the child and making a note of what the child likes to do. Another efficient procedure is to simply ask the child what he likes or what he would like to serve as a reinforcer. Any information provided voluntarily should also be acted upon immediately. Once identified, the reinforcers can be applied to appropriate behaviors to increase the frequency and/or duration that the child participates in those behaviors. If the events do not increase the level of the behavior, then one must examine the reinforcer and its application. One must determine whether the reinforcer was applied immediately enough or whether the subject was reinforced frequently enough to strengthen the response. In some cases it may be necessary to employ a shaping procedure to gradually strengthen the behavior.

Shaping is frequently used when a desired behavior is occurring at a low level or does not appear in the subject's repertoire. Shaping involves differentially reinforcing approximations of the behavior until the desired behavior or level of behavior is attained. This procedure is illustrated by the study conducted by Hanna (1971) (Case Study 3). In this study the teacher wanted to increase the number of assignments completed accurately. In order to attain this desired behavior the teacher broke the assignment into units, each containing five responses. The student was instructed to bring the paper up to the teacher's desk after he completed a unit. At that time the teacher praised the student for completing the unit and for emitting correct responses. Once the student attained what the teacher considered to be an appropriate percentage of correct responses, the size of the unit was increased to six responses. As the student was able to attain the criterion, the number was gradually increased until he was able to accurately complete the entire worksheet. Whitman, Coponigri and Mercurio (1971) also employed shaping to gradually increase the amount of time the child sat in her seat.

Thus far reinforcement has been discussed only as it pertains to increasing the strength of appropriate behaviors. In some cases, however, procedures which were implemented to decrease the frequency of behavior have had the effect of increasing the strength of the behavior. This point is well illustrated in case study 1. In Morgan (1971) the teacher continually reprimanded the student for engaging in disruptive behaviors. This served to either maintain or possibly increase the frequency of the disruptive behavior. Thus, it is conceivable that the reprimands served as reinforcers for the behavior. In fact, Morgan found that when the teacher increased the frequency of praise for appropriate behavior, a small decrease in the frequency of disruptive behavior occurred. However, when she ignored the disruptive behavior she found that there was an immediate and significant decrease in the frequency of the behavior. The same procedure was employed by Hall, Lund and Jackson (1968) to decrease disruptive behavior and increase attending behavior. Gardiner (1974) indicated the hyperactive behaviors may be strengthened by the attention provided by parents, teachers and peers. This may be particularly true if the child is ignored except when he is engaging in behaviors labeled as being hyperactive. The attention in this case may serve only to exacerbate the child's behavior, thus contributing to the development or perpetuation of the hyperactive behavior. When this occurs one procedure which can be employed to decrease the behavior is extinction.

EXTINCTION was defined by Skinner (1953) as when reinforcement is withheld and the behavior or response becomes less frequent. The decrease in the frequency will probably be dependent upon the schedule of reinforcement in use. Generally, the more intermittent the reinforcement, the more resistant the behavior is to extinction. Alternative sources of reinforcement is another variable frequently related to the effectiveness of extinction. In certain cases a parent or teacher may attempt to withhold attention for certain disruptive behaviors, but if the child's siblings or peers reinforce the behavior, extinction may not occur. Thus it is necessary to control, if possible, alternate sources of reinforcement. In addition the extinction process may be expedited if the student is concurrently reinforced for engaging in appropriate behavior. This is illustrated in Morgan (1971) (Case Study 1) and Hall, Lund and Jackson (1968).

PUNISHMENT may serve as an alternative to the use of extinction. Azrin and Holz (1966) defined punishment as "a reduction of the future probability of a specific response as a result of the immediate delivery of a stimulus for that response." This would involve applying a consequence to the target behavior. If the consequence is a punisher, the frequency of the behavior should diminish. Punishment has been found to work most efficiently when used in conjunction with other management techniques. Azrin and Holz (1966) have indicated that when punishment is combined with extinction, a rapid elimination of the target behavior is evidenced. According to Hall (1971) punishment is the fastest way to decrease the frequency of a given behavior, but he pointed out that it should be used in conjunction with reinforcement for appropriate behavior. The punishment procedure serves to reduce the strength of the inappropriate behavior while reinforcement increases the frequency of appropriate behavior. Thus, if a student is punished for leaving his seat, this doesn't necessitate an increase in academic responding. If, however, the student is reinforced for attending, correct academic responses and/or appropriate social behavior, then these behaviors should increase in frequency concurrent with the decrease in the frequency of the inappropriate behavior.

Response cost is a procedure used to reduce the frequency of a behavior. It is illustrated in Case Study 4, where students in a second grade class were required to forego one minute of recess for each disruption. The implementation of the response cost procedure correlated with a substantial decrease in the frequency of disruptive behaviors. Response cost has also been built into many token reinforcement systems to enhance the effectiveness of the system in decreasing inappropriate behavior.

Time out from positive reinforcement is yet another response reduction procedure which has been used widely. This procedure involves removing the student from the environment for a specified period of time contingent upon the student emitting an inappropriate behavior. Thus, if a child emits a disruptive behavior, he is removed to a chair facing the corner of the room, a cubicle, an isolation booth, a hallway or some other isolated area. The use of the procedure requires that the subject be in a reinforcing environment and that the removal be to a sterile environment. One variable related to the efficacy of time out has been the length of time spent in time out. White, Nielsen and Johnson (1972) compared the effects of various lengths of time out intervals. They found that the fifteen and thirty-minute periods significantly decreased the deviant behavior and that the one-minute interval varied in effectiveness depending upon whether it preceded or followed longer duration periods of time out. The authors found that when one-minute time out preceded longer duration of time out the frequency of the deviant behavior was effectively reduced. When, however, it was used after a longer duration of time out it was less effective in reducing the frequency of the target behavior. This finding tends to be significant because in many cases teachers and parents arbitrarily designate long intervals of time out, then question the efficacy of the procedure in diminishing the hyperactive behaviors emitted by their children.

ANTECEDENT EVENTS. The commentary provided so far has focused primarily upon consequent events or events that occur after the behavior is emitted. There is another area, however, which hasn't been researched quite as extensively in applied settings but which is relevant to the management of hyperactive behavior. This area has been labeled antecedent events, and it includes the events which occurred prior to the behavior being emitted. Antecedent events include instructions, seating arrangements and instructional sequences.

Instructions, according to Rieth and Hall (1974), play a very important role in the classroom. The teacher or parent uses instructions to assist in managing social behavior and to facilitate the initiation of academic activity. Hence, antecedents might increase the probability that the child will come in contact with reinforcers because of following the instructions. This would apply to both academic and social behavior and would result in a dimunition of the inappropriate social behavior and an increase in the appropriate behavior.

Seating arrangements were found by Axelrod, Hall and Tams (1972) to exert an effect on pupils' study rates. They found that when students sat in row formations, their study rates were higher than when they sat in table formations. This finding would seem relevant to providing a room arrangement to facilitate the management of behavior of a student labeled as hyperactive. Children who are highly distractible are sometimes placed in cubicles to improve their academic and attending behavior. These strategies would also increase the chance that the children would emit appropriate behavior and be reinforced. In cases where the probability of emitting appropriate behavior is increased, it is incumbent upon the person responsible for managing the children's behavior to provide the reinforcement necessary to maintain or increase the strength of the behavior. The failure to provide the reinforcement might precipitate an increase in the frequency of the undesired behaviors.

The probability of the child emitting correct academic responses can be increased by providing curricular methods and materials which are consonant with the child's academic repertoire. For example, Lovitt and Curtiss (1969) found that they could increase the rate of correct math responses emitted by an eleven-year-old by having him verbalize the problem before writing the answer. Rieth, Axelrod, Anderson, Hathaway Wood and Fitzgerald (in press) found that students did better on weekly spelling tests when they received a portion of the words each day and were tested daily. In these studies the probability that the students would be reinforced was increased by the effective manipulation of antecedent events. Another very important antecedent event is the sequence of academic materials. This would involve the selection of materials which are consonant with the student's academic repertoire. The proper selection should facilitate an increase in the probability of the student emitting correct academic responses which is basically incompatible with many of the inappropriate social behaviors listed as hyperactive. Thus, the opportunity to obtain reinforcement for appropriate behavior is greatly enhanced.

SUMMARY

This chapter has dealt with a behavioral approach to the management of hyperactive behavior. The emphasis has been placed on the presentation of procedures which have been demonstrated to effectively modify behaviors frequently ascribed to children designated as hyperactive. Though the chapter has discussed many facets of behavior management the greatest emphasis has been placed on reinforcement of appropriate behavior. It is hoped that this will serve as a model for others to emulate. The intent has been to provide an overview as well as specific illustrations of how behavioral principles can be employed to manage the behavior of children labeled as hyperactive. Nine studies are presented in the appendix to illustrate the application of behavioral principles to modify behaviors frequently listed under the rubric of hyperactivity.

CASE STUDIES

The following eight studies were conducted by educators who were enrolled in behavior management classes taught by the author. The studies were completed as a requirement of the course and demonstrate the efficacy with which educators can implement behavioral principles after being provided instruction regarding the derivation and use of the principles. The studies were selected because they illustrate the efficacy of a variety of procedures on a number of behaviors frequently described as hyperactive. The treatment procedures in some of the studies contained some confounding variables which might cause one to qualify some of the conclusions. The fact remains, however, that the educators were able to effectively implement behavioral principles in a manner that facilitates application and replication by other educators.

Case Study 1

Modifying the Disruptive Behaviors of a Third Grade Sudent

Experimenter, KATHY MORGAN

David, the Subject, was a boy nearly nine years old, enrolled in third grade. He was referred to Mrs. Morgan's remedial reading class because of unsatisfactory reading performance and low scores on the reading section of the California Reading Test. Mrs. Morgan, David and three other third graders met for thirty minutes a day. During this thirty-minute period David appeared to be in perpetual motion, emitting a number of behaviors that disrupted the group. David talked out loudly, left his seat without permission, rolled his pencil down his desk repeatedly, tapped his foot, banged the lid of his desk, flipped the pages of his book loudly and gestured to other students by waving his hand or foot. In addition, the student read very few words correctly when called upon to read orally and often looked around at the group after reading a word or words incorrectly.

BASELINE 1. During baseline the teacher recorded, during a twenty-minute period, the frequency of disruptive behaviors which encompassed all of the behaviors previously described. The twenty-minute period began five minutes after David arrived in class and continued until five minutes remained in the class.

The teacher generally reprimanded the student for all disruptions. Other interactions were relegated to feedback statements regarding the student's performance on reading tasks. During this condition David averaged 11.2 disruptive behaviors during the twenty-minute period. Reliability was 87 percent.

EXPERIMENTAL CONDITION 1 (Increased Praise). The teacher increased the frequency of praise for attending behavior while she

CASE STUDY 1

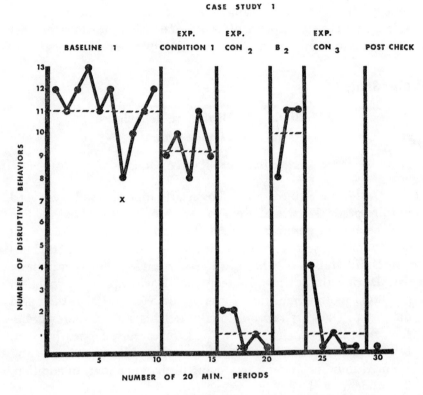

Figure 3-1.

continued to reprimand him for being disruptive. The mean number of disruptive behaviors dropped to 9.4.

EXPERIMENTAL CONDITION 2 (Increased Praise and Ignoring). During this condition all disruptive behaviors were ignored while praise was given for attending behavior. Consequently, David received attention only for appropriate behavior. A sharp decrease in the frequency of the target behavior ensued with the mean number of disruptive behaviors dropping to 1. Reliability recorded during this condition was 93.5 percent.

BASELINE 2. This condition was exactly like baseline 1. During the three days that this condition was in effect the mean number of disruptions increased to 10.

EXPERIMENTAL CONDITION 3 (Increased Praise and Ignoring). This condition was exactly the same as experimental condition 2 except for a slight dimunition of the frequency of reinforcement for attending behavior. The mean number of disruptions recorded during this condition was also 1.

POSTCHECKS. One postcheck was recorded and no disruptions were recorded. In addition, the teacher indicated that there was a correlated increase in reading achievement. The cause could not be ascertained but, most importantly, a change did occur.

Case Study 2

Increasing the Attending Behavior of a Hyperactive Child with Positive Reinforcement

Experimenter, SHARON RYAN

The subject, James, was a seven-and-one-half-year-old male who had been diagnosed by his physician as hyperkinetic and was taking Dexedrine. He had a history of having a low frustration level, talking out frequently, throwing books and running around the classroom. The frequent emittence of these behaviors precipitated his placement in a self-contained class for emotionally disturbed children. While in the special education class the running and throwing behaviors decreased, but he was observed to have a low rate of attending and a high frequency of talking to himself. His assignments were rarely finished because of his low rate of attending, frequent mumbling and playing with his pencil and other items around his desk.

For this study the student was observed while participating in a tutorial program with the experimenter. The tutoring occurred in an alcove in the hallway immediately outside the classroom.

BASELINE 1. The experimenter used interval recording to measure the percent of attending that occurred during a ten-minute observation period. The observation period was divided into 20 thirty-second observation periods. It was necessary for attending to occur for twenty out of the thirty seconds in each interval to

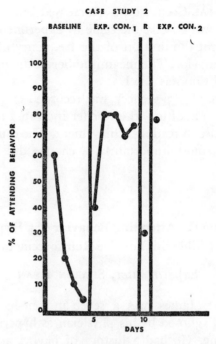

Figure 3-2.

qualify as attending behavior. Attending behavior included look-ing at the assignment, writing responses and asking questions re-lated to his work.

During baseline the student worked on individually pre-scribed reading activities while seated at his desk in the alcove. He did not receive any praise for attending or completing assignments, and attending ranged from 5 to 60 with a mean of 24 percent.

EXPERIMENTAL CONDITION 1 (Token Reinforcement). Dur-ing his condition Jim received a slip of paper with ten squares on it. He was told that each square represented a thirty-second in-terval and he would earn an X in a square for each thirty-second period of time that he paid attention. When he filled all ten squares he would be entitled to exchange it for a trinket or little toy. The trinkets or toys included a little plastic car, a balloon and a big plastic tooth. The student was also told that after filling the first slip he could earn a bonus trinket for obtaining five checks on a second slip. Consequently, the mean percent of attending during this condition rose to 70 percent.

BASELINE 2. This condition was exactly like baseline 1. The condition, however, lasted only one day because of the short summer school session. The percent of attending was 35 percent.

EXPERIMENTAL CONDITION 2 (Token Reinforcement). The token system was reinstated and was the same as experimental period 1. During this condition 82 percent attending was recorded. Due to the success of the program during the summer session, it was recommended for implementation as part of Jim's program for the regular school year.

Case Study 3

Increasing the Academic Performance of a Disruptive First Grade Student

Experimenter, GRACE HANNA

The subject, Philip, was an eight-year-old first grade student. He had been retained in first grade because of immaturity and deficient academic behavior. Mrs. Hanna noted that the student was active and that the activity was generally incompatible with accurate completion of academic assignments. Mrs. Hanna noted that the student periodically left his seat or when in his seat he would find a myriad of things in his desk or in the vicinity of his desk to play with or manipulate.

BASELINE 1. The teacher was primarily concerned with Philip's performance in phonics. Consequently she recorded the percent of correct responses achieved on daily phonics work sheets. The students were generally given four or five worksheets a day and they were done at their desks while they awaited their turn to read orally. The worksheet exercises involved filling in the missing letter or sentence completion exercises. The mean percent of correct responses was 31.

EXPERIMENTAL CONDITION 1 (Partial Worksheet). During this

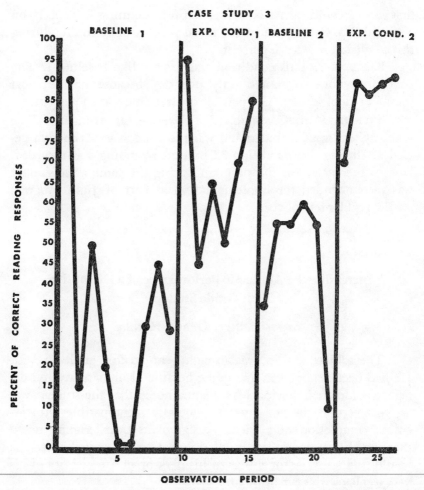

Figure 3-3.

condition the teacher divided each assignment into units and each unit encompassed five responses. The student was told that he should bring his paper to the teacher when he finished a unit. At that time the teacher checked Philip's paper and complimented the student for correct responses as well as completing the unit. The next unit was assigned and the student was asked to come to the teacher's desk when he finished the unit. In addition, the teacher also made it a point to compliment Philip periodically for sitting in his seat and attending to task. The average score achieved during this condition was 68 percent.

BASELINE 2. This condition was the same as baseline 1. The mean score recorded during this condition was 45 percent.

EXPERIMENTAL CONDITION 2 (Partial Worksheet). This condition was the same as experimental condition 1 in which the teacher had the student complete one unit of his assignment at a time. During this condition Philip averaged 86 percent on daily phonics worksheets.

DISCUSSION. The teacher indicated that as Philip's academic achievement increased there was a simultaneous decrease in the frequency of out-of-seat behavior and there was a decrease in the level of noise eminating from the vicinity of his desk. In addition, many of the playing and object manipulation behaviors were reduced in frequency. Mrs. Hanna indicated that as Philip's performance increased, she increased the number of responses in each unit. This was done in order to shape the student's repertoire so that he could eventually complete an entire worksheet before going to the teacher's desk.

Case Study 4

The Modification of the Inappropriate Behavior
of a Second Grade Student

Experimenter, MARGARET WILHELM

The subject, Rodney, was a seven-year-old student in Mrs. Wilhelm's class. He was reportedly functioning at a low second grade level in language arts and reading at a low third grade level in math. The teacher was primarily concerned, however, with Rodney's social behavior. Previously he had been labeled as hyperactive because he was out of his seat frequently and engaged in numerous talk outs.

Mrs. Wilhelm was also concerned regarding the frequency of these behaviors. She indicated to the students that they should ob-

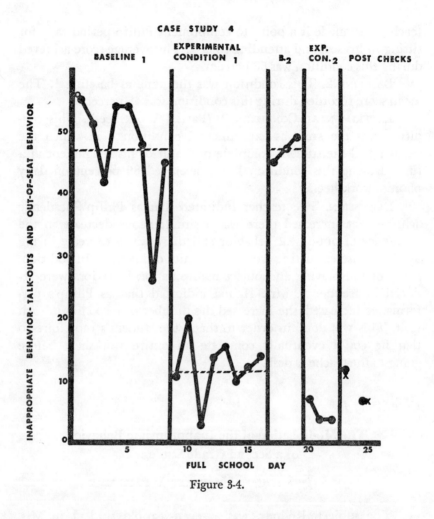

Figure 3-4.

tain teacher permission by raising their hands, and be granted permission before leaving their seats and talking out. However, Rodney persisted and consequently disturbed the class.

BASELINE 1. The teacher began to record data regarding the number of times that Rodney was out of his seat or talked out without permission in the nearly five hours of the school day spent on academic-related activities. She found that during the baseline period Rodney talked out or was out of his seat without permission forty-seven times.

EXPERIMENTAL CONDITION 1 (Rules and Consequences). During this condition a multifaceted treatment program was implemented. Initially the teacher arbitrarily divided the day into free time and quiet periods. Free time took place during art, music, game or activity time, milk time and library time. All pupils were allowed to move freely about the room, chat, sharpen pencils, get books from the library and play games. Running and yelling were not allowed. Quiet time was employed when the students were working on academic subjects including math, reading and language arts. The necessity of being quiet during academic classes was pointed out to the students. Before each session the children were informed of the rules for quiet time. The students who violated the rules for either time designation were required to stay in their seats for one minute during recess or after school, depending on when the behavior occurred. In addition, the teacher praised Rodney for emitting appropriate academic behavior. During this condition Rodney averaged a little over eleven talk outs and out-of-seats.

BASELINE 2. This condition was the same as baseline 1. During this condition Rodney averaged forty-four talk outs and out-of-seats.

EXPERIMENTAL CONDITION 2 (Rules and Consequences). This condition was the same as experimental condition 1. During the three days this condition was in effect five inappropriate behaviors were recorded.

POSTCHECKS indicated that the frequency of inappropriate behavior was remaining around nine inappropriate behaviors per five-hour recording period.

DISCUSSION. The multifaceted experimental program successfully reduced Rodney's behavior. The teacher reported that the procedure also substantially reduced the frequency of inappropriate behavior emitted by other students in class. Obviously we are unable to determine the critical variable of the many variables which were included in the treatment package. A component analysis would be recommended. The point remains, however, that the teacher was able to substantially reduce the frequency of inappropriate behavior with very little response cost.

Case Study 5

Using Group Contingencies to Modify Individual
Behavior Problems

Experimenter, RUTH GRIFFITH

The subject, Frank, was a male ten-year-old fourth grade student. He transferred to Mrs. Griffith's fourth grade class during the latter part of the first semester. He was reported by his parents to be on tranquilizers, and his prior teacher indicated that "he does a lot of moving around the classroom, or if he is in his seat he also remains in perpetual motion." In addition, the student asked to make frequent trips to the restroom and failed to pay attention to academic tasks.

Prior to Frank's arrival Mrs. Griffith reported that her class was quiet and productive. After he enrolled he attempted to obtain attention from the other students by showing off, but for the most part he was ignored. Frank then began getting out of his seat frequently and wandering around the classroom, poking other students or disturbing them in other ways. When questioned regarding the reason for being out of his seat, he indicated that he was going to sharpen his pencil or disposing of a piece of trash. The teacher indicated that he frequently talked out, which served to further disrupt the entire class. Consequently the class was in turmoil as a result of Frank's antics.

BASELINE 1. During this condition the teacher recorded the number of times Frank left his seat without permission and the number of times he talked out without permission during a three-hour period of time during the morning. During baseline Frank averaged 19.6 talk outs with a range from fourteen to thirty-two and 11.1 out-of-seats with a range from five to sixteen.

EXPERIMENTAL CONDITION 1 (Good behavior game). The teacher introduced the good behavior game (Barrish, Saunders,

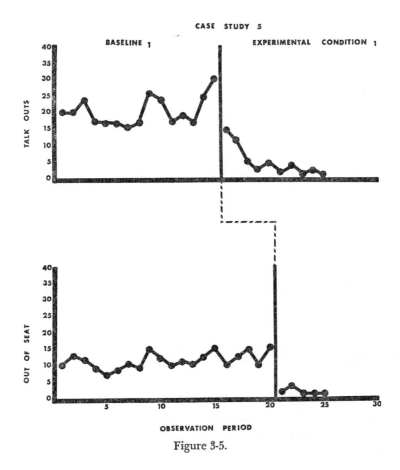

Figure 3-5.

and Wolf, 1969). The students in the class were told "Since three new students moved in there is less room to move about in the classroom and if everyone started to walk around or to talk the noise would be so great that no one could study." The students were instructed that if they wanted to talk or get out of their seats it would be necessary to obtain teacher permission. Permission was obtained by raising their hands and requesting permission.

The good behavior game involved dividing the room in half and designating each half as a team. The teacher then indicated that each team would be penalized one point any time one of its members talked out without permission. Each team was allowed five talk outs. If they had less than five the team would have free time to play games during the last thirty minutes of the school day. During this condition Frank averaged 7.8 talk outs per observation period. The number ranged from three to fourteen with the lower number of behaviors occurring a few days after the contingency was applied. When the teams were regularly attaining the criteria, the teacher then indicated out-of-seats would also be counted. This meant that a total of five out-of-seats and talk outs were allowed. A total above this number meant that the team did not get the free time and was required to begin working on their homework. As a result of the introduction of this part of the contingency, Frank's average number of talk outs dropped to 1.4 and the number of out-of-seats to .6.

DISCUSSION. The results show that group consequences could be used to modify the behavior of an individual student as well as the class. The teacher noted that Frank was less active, quieter, finished more academic tasks and completed them more accurately when the good behavior game was in effect.

Case Study 6

The Use of Good Worker Seat Covers to Decrease the Frequency of Talk Out and Out of Seat Behaviors

Experimenter, GRACE HANNA

Mrs. Hanna, a first grade teacher, was concerned regarding the behavior of her twenty-two-student first grade class. She was concerned regarding the noise in the class and the frequency of movement around the classroom. In particular, she was concerned regarding the behavior of one particular female student. The girl, Jill, would impulsively talk out, she was frequently out of her seat, she would crawl under her desk or around the classroom on the floor or she would frequently sprawl out on top of her desk.

The teacher recorded the number of talk outs and out-of-seats occurring in the class during a two-hour observation period. Talk

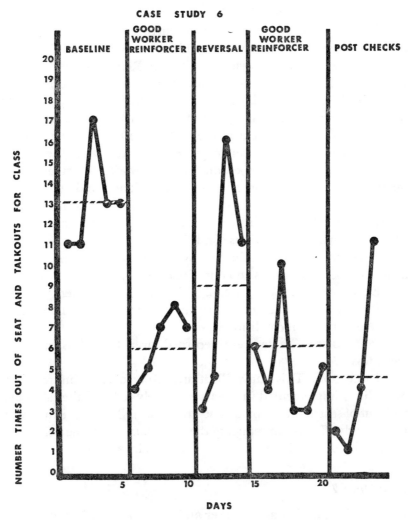

Figure 3-6.

outs were defined as speaking out before raising a hand and being recognized. Out-of-seats were defined as being absent from an assigned chair for reasons other than the participation in a reading group, taking completed work papers to the collection basket or getting a Kleenex®.

BASELINE 1. During baseline 1 the teacher recorded the number of talk outs and out-of-seats occurring during a two-hour period of time during the morning. The mean was 13.

EXPERIMENTAL CONDITION 1 (Token Reinforcement). Each student was given five tokens, which were plastic discs, to keep on top of his/her desk. During the two-hour reading period a token was lost for each talk out or out-of-seat. Each student, however, who retained all five tokens at the end of the two-hour period received a Good Worker cover to put on the back of his/her chair and a smile face was stamped on the good worker chart opposite the student's name. The mean number of talk outs and out-of-seats was reduced to 6. The target student only had one talk out or out-of-seat recorded during this condition. A drop from an average of 6 per day during the previous condition.

BASELINE 2. This condition was the same as baseline 1. The mean number of talk outs and out of seats was 9.

EXPERIMENTAL CONDITION 2 (Token Reinforcement). This condition was the same as in experimental condition 1. The mean recorded during this condition was 6.

POSTCHECKS. These were recorded over four days and the mean was 4.5.

DISCUSSION. This study illustrates how token reinforcement procedures implemented in a class effectively reduced the talk outs and out-of-seat emitted by a first grade class. The procedure was particularly effective in reducing the frequency that those behaviors were emitted by a girl who had been labeled hyperactive.

Case Study 7

The Teacher as Observer and Experimenter in the Modification of Talking Out Behavior

Experimenter, CARROLL TUCKER

The subject, Ted, was an eight-year-old third grade pupil. He was reportedly capable of being an excellent student, but because of disruptive behavior he had achieved less than satisfactory grades. Mrs. Tucker indicated that Ted was constantly disturbing

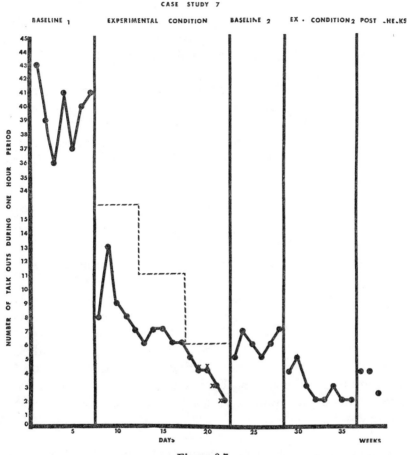

Figure 3-7.

others with his unauthorized talk outs. He frequently ridiculed other students which provoked fights, he interrupted conversations between students and talked with other students while the teacher was giving directions for assignments. These behaviors were generally incompatible with accurate completion of assigned academic work.

BASELINE 1. During baseline the teacher recorded the number of talk outs recorded during the first hour of the school day. During this hour the class worked on reading activities, discussed daily assignments, conducted opening exercises and had music twice a week. Generally during this condition the teacher reprimanded Ted when she felt he was talking too much or if he was involved in an altercation. The number of talk outs ranged from thirty-six to forty-three will a median of forty.

EXPERIMENTAL CONDITION 1 (Chain Links). At the beginning of this condition the teacher repeated the rules regarding the necessity of obtaining permission before talking out. Ted was told initially that if he talked out less than fifteen times he would earn a paper link that would serve as part of a paper chain. Each link earned had a clever saying written on it. Ted was told that when he earned fifteen links he would earn a bottle of pop and a candy bar. During the five-day period the criterion was in effect the number of talk outs ranged from seven to thirteen. When the criterion was diminished to ten the subject met the criterion every day. The median number of talk outs recorded during this section was eight. Next, the criterion was lowered to five, and the subject responded by lowering his median number of talk outs to four. Reliability checks conducted during this condition yielded a mean of 100 percent.

BASELINE 2. After Ted earned his bottle of pop and candy bar the teacher told him that he was doing so well that it wouldn't be necessary to use the system. The condition was the same as baseline 1. The median number of talk outs recorded during this condition was six.

EXPERIMENTAL CONDITION 2 (Chain Link). This condition was the same as experimental condition 1. The talk out limit was five and the reinforcer for staying below the limit for eight consecutive days was a bar of candy. The median number of talk outs recorded during this condition was four.

POSTCHECKS. Postchecks were made at one-week intervals over a three-week period. The talk outs remained at a low level despite the fact that reinforcement was discontinued.

Case Study 8

The Principal as a Behavior Management Specialist

Experimenter, CHARLES ANDERSON

Carl was a male third grader at Indian Creek School, located in a middle class community in the county area surrounding Topeka, Kansas. Carl was of average intelligence but attained achievement test scores which were approximately one year below his grade level placement. His greatest fame was achieved as a result of his social behavior.

Carl's antics were one of the favorite topics for discussion in the teacher's lounge. These antics were mainly in the area of talkouts. He disputed and argued with the teacher. He yelled at, talked to and argued with his peers. Carl also spent a considerable amount of time moving around the classroom. This tended to increase the number of verbal and physical conflicts which occurred. In addition, the teacher was concerned about Carl's academic performance, particularly in arithmetic.

Carl's teacher was so frustrated by his behavior that she requested that the principal place him in a class for the emotionally disturbed. At the time of the request the personnel necessary to make the placement were unavailable, therefore the principal suggested that he and the teacher plan a program for Carl. He said he would visit the class to observe and/or assist the teacher in recording data.

The three behaviors recorded were talkouts, attending behavior and the percent of correct arithmetic responses.

TALKOUTS were defined as sounds, audible to the teacher, emitted by Carl without explicit teacher permission. This behavior was recorded by the teacher during the thirty-minute arithmetic period. The teacher made a tally on a slip of paper which she always carried with her when a talk out was observed.

ATTENDING was defined as looking at the assignment sheet or work materials. In addition, any contact with the teacher such as raising his/her hand for help or discussion of the assignment was counted as attending. In-group attending was defined as orienta-

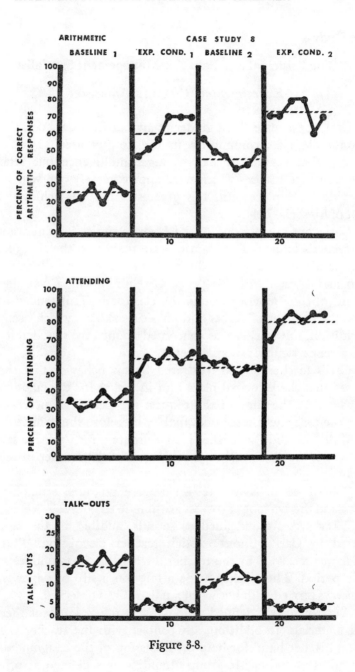

Figure 3-8.

tion toward work materials, to a reciting fellow student, to the teacher or, if responding orally, to a lesson. Time sample recording was used to measure this behavior.

PERCENT OF CORRECT ARITHMETIC RESPONSES were calculated by dividing the number of problems answered correctly by the number of problems assigned. These data were collected by the teacher. Reliability was provided by the principal, who made simultaneous independent recordings.

BASELINE 1. During this condition, the teacher and principal observed and recorded independently the percent of attending, percent of correct arithmetic responses, and the number of talkouts.

The lesson format consisted of the teacher presenting the lecture material and a demonstration of solution strategies with sample problems. The students were then assigned problems to solve. The mean percent of correct responses was 26 percent, the mean percent of attending was 35 percent, and the mean number of talk outs was sixteen.

EXPERIMENTAL CONDITION 1 (Token Reinforcement 1). The teacher and principal devised a token reinforcement system which the teacher implemented. The tokens consisted of construction paper discs of three different colors. Carl earned a red disc for each correct answer. When five problems were worked correctly, Carl earned a blue disc and he earned a gold disc for ten correctly-answered problems. The discs were traded for stars of the same color that were pasted on a wall chart next to the student's name. In addition, a gold disc earned an animal stamp which was placed on the top of his paper. During this condition, the mean percent of correct arithmetic responses increased to 62 percent while the mean percent of attending increased to 59 percent and the mean number of talk outs decreased to four.

BASELINE II. The procedures were the same as those in Baseline I. When baseline conditions were reintroduced the mean percent of correct arithmetic responses dropped to 45 percent, the mean percent of attending decreased slightly to 53 percent and the mean number of talk outs rose to 12.

EXPERIMENTAL CONDITION 2 (Token Reinforcement). This condition was the same as Token Reinforcement I with the exception of the addition of a piece of penny candy earned for each gold token disc. When the modified token system was implemented, the mean percent of correct math responses rose to 72 percent, the mean percent of attending increased to 72 percent, and the mean number of talkouts decreased to four.

DISCUSSION. The data collected documented the effectiveness of the program devised by the principal and the teacher. The token system implemented by the teacher was simple and effective, yet relatively cost-free. The only cost was the price of a few penny candy bars used as back-up reinforcers. The purpose was to facilitate a substantial increase in the arithmetic scores. Once this was accomplished, the stars were used for maintenance. In addition, it should be noted that the effects of the token system generalized to both attending behavior and talk outs.

Because of the token system's success, it was implemented in other subject areas with comparable success. This success caused the teacher to continue the system until the end of the school year.

The principal reported that prior to the next school year he conferred with the teacher and suggested the use of differential reinforcement to maintain the gains attained during the previous year. In fact, data collected by the principal at the end of Carl's fourth grade year indicated that his achievement test scores were commensurate with his grade level placement. In addition, the teacher was reportedly very complimentary of Carl's appropriate social behavior.

Thus, because of the initial intervention on the part of the principal and the teacher, the student's behavior was changed. This avoided the necessity of placing the student in a high cost special education class and spared the student the ignominy of being segregated in a special class. We found, also, that the teacher acquired skills which were valuable additions to her repertoire. Consequently, these skills would also benefit other students with whom the teacher had contact.

REFERENCES

Anderson, C.: The Principal as a Behavior Management Specialist. Unpublished manuscript, University of Kansas, 1972.

Axelrod, S., Hall, R.V., and Tams, A.: A Comparison of Two Common Seating Arrangements in Classroom Settings. Paper presented at the third annual meeting of the Kansas Symposium on Behavior Analysis in Education, Lawrence, Kansas, May, 1972.

Azrin, N.H., and Holz, W.C.: Punishment. In Honig, W.K. (Ed.): *Operant Behavior: Areas of Research and Application.* New York, Appleton, 1966.

Baer, D.M., Wolf, M.M., and Risley, T.R.: Some current dimensions of applied behavior analysis. *J Appl Beh Anal, 1:*91-97, 1968.

Barrish, H.H., Saunders, M., and Wolf, M.M.: Good behavior game: Effects of individual contingencies for group consequences on disruptive behavior in a classroom. *J Appl Beh Anal, 2:*119-124, 1969.

Bijou, S.W., and Baer, D.M.: *Child Development I: A Systematic and Empirical Theory.* New York, Appleton, 1961.

Boyle, J.P.: Psychophysiological Support for Differentiated Diagnosis in the Hyperactivity Syndrome. Unpublished manuscript, University of Northern Colorado, 1974.

Cooper, J.O.: *Measurement and Analysis of Behavioral Techniques.* Columbus, Merrill, 1974.

Cruickshank, W.M.: *The Brain-Injured Child in Home, School and Community.* Syracuse, Syracuse U Pr, 1967.

Doubros, S.G., and Daniels, G.J.: An experimental approach to the reduction of overactive behavior. *Beh Res Ther, 4:*251-258, 1966.

Gardner, W.I.: *Children With Learning and Behavior Problems: A Behavior Management Approach.* Boston, Allyn, 1974.

Griffith, R.: Using Group Contingencies to Modify Individual Behavior Problems. Unpublished manuscript, University of Kansas, 1971.

Hall, R.V.: *Managing behavior.* Lawrence, H & H Enterprises, Inc., vol. 1-3, 1971.

Hall, R.V., Lund, D., and Jackson, D.: Effects of teacher attention on study behavior. *J Appl Beh Anal, 1:*1-12, 1968.

Hanna, G.: Increasing the Academic Performance of a Disruptive First Grade Student. Unpublished manuscript, University of Kansas, 1971.

Hanna, G.: The Use of Good Worker Seat Covers to Decrease the Frequency of Talk Out and Out of Seat Behaviors. Unpublished manuscript, University of Kansas, 1972.

Hoffman, H.: *The Story of Fidgety Philip* (1844). Translated by Mann, G. New York, Dover, 1970.

Keogh, B.K.: Hyperactivity and learning disorders: Review and speculation. *Except Child, 38:*101-109, 1971.

Keogh, B.K.: Hyperactivity and learning problems: Implications for teachers. *Ed Dig, 37:*45-47, 1971.

Lovitt, T.C., and Curtiss, K.A.: Effects of manipulating and antecedent event on mathematics response rate. *J Appl Beh Anal, 1*:329-333, 1969.

Morgan, K.: Modifying the Disruptive Behaviors of a Third Grade Student. Unpublished manuscript, University of Kansas, 1971.

Patterson, G.R.: A Tentative Approach to the Classification of Childrens Behavior Problems. Unpublished doctoral dissertation, University of Minnesota, 1955.

Patterson, G.R.: An application of conditioning techniques to the control of a hyperactive child. In Ullman, L.P., and Krasner, L. (Ed.): *Case Studies in Behavior Modification.* New York. H R & W, 1966, pp. 370-375.

Rieth, H.J.: Experimental Analysis of Procedures Used to Modify the Academic and Attending Behavior of Students Alternately Placed in Regular and Special Education. Unpublished doctoral dissertation, University of Kansas, 1971.

Rieth, H.J., Axelrod, S., Anderson, R., Hathaway, F., Wood, K., and Fitzgerald, C.: Influence of distributed practice and daily testing on weekly spelling tests. *J Ed Res,* In press.

Rieth, H.J., and Hall, R.V.: *Responsive teaching model readings in applied behavior analysis.* Lawrence, H&H Enterprises, 1974.

Risley, T.R.: Spontaneous language in the preschool environment. In Julian Stanley (Ed.): *Preschool Programs for the Disadvantaged.* Baltimore, John Hopkins, 1972.

Ryan, S.: Increasing the attending behavior of a hyperactive child with positive reinforcement. Unpublished manuscript, University of Missouri-St. Louis, 1971.

Schmitt, B.D., Martin, H.P., Nellhaus, G., Cravens, J., Camp, B.W., and Jordan, K.: The hyperactive child. *Clin Pediatr, 12*:154-169, 1973.

Sidman, M.: *Tactics of Scientific Research.* New York, Basic, 1960.

Skinner, B.F.: *Science and Human Behavior.* New York, Free Pr, 1953.

Sulzer, B., and Mayer, G.R.: *Behavior Modification Procedures for School Personnel.* Hinsdale, Dryden Press, 1972.

Tucker, C.: The Teacher as Observer and Experimenter in the Modification of Talking Out Behavior. Unpublished manuscript, University of Kansas, 1973.

Werry, J.S., Klaus, M., Guzman, A., Weiss, G., Dogan, K., and Hoy, E.: Studies on the hyperactive child — VII: neurological status compared with neurotic and normal children. *Am J Orthopsychiatry, 42*:44-54, 1972.

White, G.D., Nielsen, G., and Johnsen, S.M.: Timeout duration and the suppression of deviant behavior in children. *J Appl Beh Anal, 5*:111-120, 1972.

Whitman, T.Y., Caponegri, V., and Mercurio, J.: Reducing hyperactive behavior in a severely retarded child. *Ment Retard, 9*:17-19, 1971.

Wilhelm, M.: The Modification of the Inappropriate Behaviors of a Second Grade Student. Unpublished manuscript, University of Kansas, 1972.

4

Educational management of hyperactive children

Norma J. Dyck

T HIS CHAPTER FOCUSES on the educational management of hyperactive children. The primary concern is with the
relationship of hyperactive behavior to school and learning problems and how to deal with these problems in the school environment. Controlling hyperactive behavior to facilitate the child's
social adjustment is important but is not addressed in this discussion. More definitively, this chapter focuses on the educational
management of a child when hyperactivity, distractibility, inattentiveness or impulsivity appears to interfere with learning.

A discussion of the topic requires an operational definition
of *hyperactive children* since the term has been used to describe
children with emotional disturbance, brain damage, environmental deprivation and other categorical descriptions. Werry
(1968) defined hyperactivity as "a total daily motor activity (or
movement of the body or any portion of it) which is significantly
greater than the norm (p. 581)." Such a definition does not imply
causation and is useful for this discussion.

The need for special educational planning for hyperactive
children is well documented. The exact nature of the learning

problems and factors related to them are less explicit. Werry (1968) hypothesized two sources of learning problems among hyperactive children—the reduced amount of time spent on a learning task, and cognitive disorders such as visual-motor deficits which interfere with learning in a normal classroom curriculum.

More recently, Keogh (1971) proposed three hypotheses to explain the relationships and interactions of hyperactivity and learning problems. The hypotheses were not seen as exhaustive or mutually exclusive, and each had implications for different remedial approaches and treatment plans.

The first hypothesis referred to a medical explanation. Learning problems, distractibility, perceptual problems and motor hyperactivity were perceived as symptoms all caused by neurological impairment. When hyperactive behavior is explained in this manner, the corrective measures attempt to remove the cause rather than deal directly with the learning problem and related symptoms. For example, medication can be prescribed, and it apparently affects the neurological system in such a way that the behavioral and learning symptoms are controlled or minimized. Subjects related to medical interventions are presented in the chapter by Myra and Reece.

Some advocates of perceptual-motor training (Delacato, 1959 and Kephart, 1960) attempt to control or change the neurological dysfunction, using gross motor activities, on the theory that the physical training will benefit both perception and learning of school tasks. The effectiveness of these perceptual-motor activities in improving the academic learning of hyperactive children is inconclusive. Werry (1968) cautioned,

> The efflorescence of the nonmedical professionals offering "perceptual-motor training" should be viewed with a skepticism proper to all new treatment methods until scientifically impeccable data attest to its value. Readers are reminded also that any relationship between dominance, motor coordination and body image on the one hand and reading, writing and arithmetic on the other is, in the present state of knowledge, pure speculation (p. 593).

In a later document, Hammill (1975) also encouraged caution when he wrote,

Because perceptual-motor programs are currently much in vogue, thousands of elementary, special education, and preschool teachers base their readiness, preventive, and corrective activities exclusively or in part on such programs. . . . Teachers should be urged to implement perceptual-motor training on a remedial basis in only those few cases where improvement in perception is the goal and to consider such efforts as experimental. The efficacy of providing training to all children has not been sufficiently demonstrated to warrant the expenditure of the school's funds or the teacher's time. In general, perceptual-motor training is viewed as more acceptable for preschool than for kindergarten or school-aged children, and is never recommended as a substitute for teaching language, reading, or arithmetic skills (p. 230).

Since the effectiveness of perceptual-motor training programs for hyperactive children is equivocal, this intervention approach will not be discussed in detail in this chapter. Thorough descriptions of theory and application of perceptual-motor training programs are written by Kephart (1960), Getman, Kane, Halgren and McKee (1968), Barsch (1965) and Delacato (1959).

The second hypothesis advanced by Keogh (1971) described the learning problems of the hyperactive child in this way: the nature and extent of his/her motor activity disrupt the accurate acquisition of information. When this hypothesis is applied, intervention approaches might include securing the child's attention at the information acquisition stages of problem solving and controlling his/her motor activity. Behavioral modification techniques and/or medication have been effective in control of attention and motor activity. These methods have been credited with improving learning among some hyperactive children. Principles of behavioral management are discussed in the chapter by Rieth. Some applications of these principles in the educational program are also included in this chapter.

Strauss and Lehtinen (1947) and Cruickshank and his associates (Cruickshank, Bentzen, Ratzanburg and Tannhauser, 1961) proposed a teaching method that reduced environmental stimulation, increased the stimulus value of instructional materials and removed extraneous stimuli from the materials. This method was designed to help focus the child's attention on the critical elements of information. Portions of this method will be explained in this chapter.

Finally, Keogh (1971) hypothesized that learning problems of hyperactive children may be a function of hasty, impulsive decisions in the learning situation. With this explanation, intervention techniques can be recommended that emphasize helping the child slow down when making critical decisions. There is some evidence that teaching approaches which employ overt speech controls (Luria, 1961; Meichenbaum and Goodman, 1969 and Schwebel, 1966) or direct reinforcement of reflective behavior (Kagan, 1966; Allen, Henke, Harris, Baer, and Reynolds, 1967) may result in improved learning for hyperactive children. Yando and Kagan (1968) offered further evidence that a teacher with a reflective teaching style provides a model that is beneficial to impulsive students. Much of the work related to impulsivity and reflectivity is reported in the chapter by Wright and Vlietstra.

Although research has not provided conclusive guidelines for educators, one basic theme appears consistently in the literature on educational management of hyperactive children. The theme is *structure*. Hyperactive children, regardless of the etiology of the problem, appear to profit from highly structured environments, time, activities, rewards and tasks. Although there are variations of the theme of structure, the concept appears with persistence and forms the primary basis for educational management of hyperactive children.

The remainder of this chapter will present a discussion of educational models that have influenced the majority of special educational programs for hyperactive children. It will also present an expansion of the concepts related to structure in educational planning. The final section will offer a summary and recommendations for future educational planning for hyperactive children.

EDUCATIONAL MODELS

Special class models have dominated educational programs for hyperactive children during the past twenty-five years. For example, a structured classroom model was developed and studied by Strauss, Lehtinen (1947) and Cruickshank (1961). In addition, an example of a special class model applying behavioral modification techniques was evaluated by Hewett (1968). Since these two special class models, or aspects of them, have had a major influence on educational planning for hyperactive children, they are summarized in this chapter.

During the past decade, educators have questioned the value of special class placement as the courts are requiring children to be taught in the "least restrictive environment." New models are emerging which modify the principles of the special class models, and applications of the principles are applied in regular classrooms and resource rooms. A few examples of alternative models are cited in this discussion.

The Strauss-Lehtinen-Cruickshank Model

The most comprehensive study of educational planning specifically for hyperactive children was reported by Cruickshank and his associates in 1961. Procedures for the experimental model were based on the theoretical position of Strauss and the instructional program recommended by Lehtinen (Strauss and Lehtinen, 1947). Although the Strauss-Lehtinen program was created for children who were described as brain-injured, one of the principle characteristics of this population was hyperactivity. Therefore, much of the teaching methodology was directed toward control of the hyperactive and distractible characteristics readily apparent among the children sampled.

Having less concern for the diagnosis of brain-injury, Cruickshank et al. (1961) selected for their sample hyperactive and distractible children with or without brain injury. Additionally, the sample selected by this team consisted of children with normal or near normal intelligence in a public school setting. The following characteristics were identified among the children included in the population:

1. distractibility
2. motor disinhibition
3. dissociation

4. disturbance of figure-background relationships
5. perseveration
6. absence of a well-developed self-concept and body-image concept

Hyperactivity as defined for the study implied more than subtle deviations in behavior. It included problems of short attention span, visual and auditory distractibility, and "disturbances in perception leading to dissociative tendencies (p. 10)."

On the assumption that the cause of hyperactivity could not be removed or, in the case of emotional disturbance, that modification would be a slow process, an educational program was designed with students completely removed from normal children. The primary elements of the educational design included

* 1. reduced environmental stimuli
2. reduced space
3. a structured school program and life plan
4. an increase in the stimulus value of the teaching materials which are constructed to cope with the specific characteristics of the psychopathology under consideration

To reduce unessential environmental stimuli a room was provided in which bulletin boards, pictures and other extraneous objects had been removed. The color of the walls, woodwork and furniture matched the floor color, and windows were covered or opaqued. The room sound was carefully controlled. A well-qualified teacher was employed; she dressed in plain clothes without jewelry or other ornamental objects that might gain undue attention from the children. Space was reduced by using cubicles or placing the child in a corner or behind cabinets.

Many interesting techniques were devised, using color to control the stimulus value of visual instructional materials. Distractions such as pictures were removed from books, and color cues were added to focus attention on critical elements. For example, each numeral in an arithmetic problem might be written with a different colored ink.

The instructional program was individualized, providing opportunities for success. It involved manipulation of activities to facilitate conditioning through small sequential steps. Assignments were tailored to meet the attention span of each individual child, and daily schedules were rigidly enforced.

The curriculum stressed readiness and/or academic skill areas, rather than content areas such as social studies. Multisensory techniques and perceptual-motor tasks were incorporated into the academic learning program. Manipulative aids were employed in moving students from the concrete to the abstract. The basic principles for reading instruction included movement from parts to wholes, including an emphasis on meaning.

Cruickshank et al. (1961) believed learning was a result of perception and conditioning. The hyperactive child with a perceptual disorder experienced many failures in the school environment resulting in negative reinforcement. Based on this philosophy, Cruickshank et al. (1961) stated, "Learning and growth in the hyperactive child will be disorganized and disintegrated because distractibility prevents the perception of responses deemed socially appropriate to given stimuli." An important component of the program then required programming that provided success initially. Success became possible with gradual introduction of new concepts or associations through a conditioning process.

At the end of one year the children in the experimental classroom were compared to a control group who had received traditional special-class educational programs. The experimental group made significant gains on six of ten scoring categories of the Bender-Gestalt test. They gained significantly on the number of correct figures of the Syracuse Visual Figure Background Test and in ability to withstand distraction from background stimuli. No significant differences between groups were reported on IQ or on social development as measured by the Vineland Scale. Academic achievement was not evaluated. A follow-up study one year later, after subjects from both groups experienced educational programs completely different from the experimental plan, indicated the experimental group had lost the gains found during the earlier testing. These results suggested that the experimental program was moderately successful.

In a current summary and analysis of the results of the study, Hallahan and Cruickshank (1973) recognized the limitations of the study and advocated cautious interpretation or generalization of the results. Based on this study and other experimental evidence the authors concluded, "Meanwhile, evidence does suggest that the Strauss-Lehtinen-Cruickshank procedures benefit the perceptual and perceptual-motor ability of hyperactive and distractible children [Cruickshank et al., 1961] and that reduction of stimuli through the use of cubicles results in better attending behaviors of these children [Shores and Haubrich, 1969] and increased academic performance [Gorton, 1972] (p. 242)."

When Myers and Hammill (1969) summarized the Cruickshank et al. (1961) methods and techniques, they suggested that a program which combined the Strauss-Lehtinen-Cruickshank procedures with those of Hewett (1968) might be more effective than either model used alone. This writer concurs.

The Engineered Classroom Model

Hewett (1968) designed a special class program for children with learning and behavioral problems which resembled the Strauss-Lehtinen-Cruickshank program in many ways, but he added the use of behavioral modification techniques. In addition, a set of behavioral objectives was developed to facilitate a transition from diagnosis to educational programming. As the term *engineered classroom* implies, the teacher manipulated the classroom environment to create opportunities for positive reinforcement of appropriate educational and behavioral performance of each student.

The term *emotionally disturbed* was used to describe the population of the study. The term referred to children who were "inattentive, withdrawn, aggressive, nonconforming, disorganized, immature, and unable to get along with others . . ." (Hewett, 1968). Hewett believed there was considerable overlap that existed between the "brain-injured" syndrome described by Struass-Lehtinen-Cruickshank and the "emotionally disturbed" population of his interest. He observed that hyperactivity and distractibility were characteristics common to both categorical descriptions of children.

The classroom environment of the engineered classroom was highly organized and individualized, with many elements common to the environment recommended in the Strauss-Lehtinen-Cruickshank model. Hewett (1968) did not believe the removal of all distracting stimuli and creation of a nonstimulating environment was essential to the learning situation. "What may be more important than the physical arrangement is the manner in which assignments are made and expected behavioral standards presented to the students (p. 162)." The physical conditions believed important were room size, student desk arrangement and provision for various activity centers including study booths. Students were seated farther apart than in normal classrooms and used larger desks and sometimes tables for independent work. The larger work space was helpful since it permitted the teachers to sit down beside the students as they worked together on a learning task.

The model for the engineered classroom stressed the following instructional methodology (Hewett, 1968 p. 240):

1. Start where the child is and get him ready for more complex tasks through assignment of basic readiness tasks.

2. Settle for "thimbleful" of accomplishment and resist preoccupation with a "bucket" orientation in learning.

3. Once you have established contact with a child, gradually increase demands and expectations at a pace which the child can tolerate.

4. Attempt to guarantee that the child will experience continual success in the classroom.

5. Create a predictable learning environment for the child in which he is rewarded for his accomplishment, nonrewarded if he fails to meet demands which, according to everything known about him, are reasonable to expect of him.

6. Be prepared to back up, modify tasks, and reset expectations if the child fails.

After deconditioning the child to negative attitudes toward school and learning, a program that was planned around specific educational objectives was introduced. The teacher assessed the student's behavior using a developmental sequence of educational goals. Hewett (1972, pp. 402-403) summarized these goals in the following manner:

1. Attention
   a. Does the child pay attention to visual, auditory, and tactual stimuli associated with learning tasks given him?
   b. Does the child attend to reality events instead of fantasy?
   c. Does the child pay attention to behavior associated with assignments in the classroom or is he preoccupied with compulsive, ritualistic acts such as excessive handwashing or pencil sharpening?
   d. Has the child developed accurate beliefs about himself and the environment and does he manifest interests that are appropriate for his age and sex?
   e. Does the child pay attention to the teacher?
   f. Does the child retain directions and information given him and profit from such instruction?

2. Response
   a. Will the child freely undertake an assignment given him?
   b. Is the child constricted in his performance in the classroom and unwilling to do more than a limited amount in relation to an assignment?
   c. Does the child display a broad range of interests in subject matter and activities in the classroom?
   d. Does the child withdraw from contact with teacher and peers?
   e. Can the child function in a regular class setting or does he need a special class placement or individual tutoring?

3. Order
   a. Does the child follow directions and start, follow through, and complete assignments in the manner prescribed?
   b. Is the child impulsive and uncritical in his attempts to do assignments given him?
   c. Does the child respect the working rights of others or is he disruptive in a class group?

4. Exploratory
   a. Does the child have accurate knowledge about his environment and does he freely and thoroughly engage in multisensory exploration of it?
   b. Is the child dependent on the directions and choices of others in selecting interests and activities?
   c. Is there any evidence of motor, physical, sensory, perceptual, or intellectual deficits that limit the child's capacity to freely and accurately explore the environment?

5. Social

   a. In general, does the child's behavior gain the approval of others and avoid their disapproval?

   b. Is the child overly dependent on obtaining attention and praise from others?

6. Mastery

   a. Has the child acquired the ability to take care of himself and has he mastered cognitive and academic skills commensurate with his intellectual capacity?

7. Achievement

   a. Is the child self-motivated in learning and does he give evidence of being rewarded by acquisition of knowledge and skill?

Based on the results of the assessment, the teacher selected the lowest level of the developmental sequence in which the child was having difficulty and related it to a specific task. The expectations were clearly described to the child, and the teacher arranged the instructional task to provide opportunity for success. When successful completion occurred, a meaningful reward was given. The teaching strategy became one of constant manipulation of the stimuli and consequences.

The classroom was divided into three major centers which paralleled the levels on the developmental sequence: the "mastery-center," the "exploratory-center" and the "order center."

The "mastery-center" included student and teacher desks. Academic work was completed in this area. Two study booths were provided for completion of assignments free from distractions when the need was perceived by the student or teacher. The booths were not intended to be used in the same manner that Strauss-Lehtinen-Cruickshank encouraged. They were attractive and comfortable, simply an opportunity to be removed from visual and auditory distractions of the classroom.

The second center, "exploratory center," had three subareas and was located near the windows and a sink. One subarea provided equipment for science experiments, another contained arts and crafts activities, and the third provided a communication area containing group listening activities and games.

The third center was called the "order center" although it also included activities related to attention and response. This center contained puzzles, exercises and materials designed to enhance attending behavior and activities for following directions.

Rejecting the hypothesis of a need for a drab, sterile, nonstimulating environment, the use of three bulletin boards in the classroom was recommended. The first was used to display student work when completed, and the second contained daily work packets. The third bulletin board contained Work Record Cards displaying check marks that could be exchanged for tangible rewards.

A four-hour class schedule was rigidly enforced. A ten-minute order period was followed by an hour reading period, a ten-minute recess, a one-hour arithmetic period, a nutrition period, a physical education period and an hour of exploratory activities. As the child successfully completed activities within the guidelines provided by the teacher, he/she was given check marks on his/her Work Record Card while the teacher verbalized the reason he/she did or did not get the total possible number of check marks for that activity. At the end of the week completely filled Work Record Cards were exchanged for tangible rewards such as candy, toys or classroom privileges.

The engineered classroom model was evaluated in the Santa Monica Schools in California (Hewett, Taylor, and Artuso, 1967). Six classrooms were formed and nine children with learning or behavioral problems were assigned to each. The teacher for each classroom was trained to use the engineered classroom techniques. The experimental classrooms maintained rigid adherence to the engineered classroom design. The control classrooms were permitted to use any teaching strategy, including concepts of the engineered classroom, but they could not use check marks and tangible rewards. One classroom used the experimental condition for the entire school year while another used the control condition for the same length of time. Two classrooms used the experimental condition for the first half of the school year, then switched to the control condition; two other classrooms reversed the arrangement. The latter two classrooms began the school year with the control condition and switched to the experimental condition at the end of the semester.

The dependent variables were *task attention* and academic achievement. The only academic area favoring the experimental classroom was arithmetic, but task attention definitely favored the experimental approach. In a second study (Hewett, 1972), thirty classes of elementary students matched on age, sex, and IQ were tested on achievement gains over a one-year period. The students were placed into three groups: educationally handicapped children in an engineered classroom, educationally handicapped children in regular classrooms, and normal children in regular classrooms. The reading and arithmetic gains for children in the engineered classrooms were significantly greater than gains of the educationally handicapped children left in the regular classrooms.

On the basis of the two studies Hewett (1972 p. 410) concluded,

> In summary, the engineered classroom design appears to be particularly effective in 'launching' children with behavior disorders into learning and more actively involving them in attention, responding, and direction following. Once an investment is made in establishing these basic competencies, the child actually moves on to higher levels of the developmental sequence where he is more susceptible to approaches using exploratory, social, and mastery emphases.

Both Cruickshank and Hewett advocated placement of hyperactive children in these special classes to initiate an intervention program. They further proposed returning the student to the normal school environment as soon as a successful learning pattern was well established. Far too often this reintegration does not occur in public school settings—once children are placed in special classrooms, they remain there until they reach high school age. The problem of integrating students back into the normal classroom environment was not considered by either author. This issue is gaining attention among contemporary educators who are looking for new models of educational planning for children with learning and behavioral problems.

Alternative Models

Placement in a special classroom is a drastic measure that should be reserved for children with profound handicaps. Many hyperactive children should be taught in the normal mainstream of education. Many of the concepts presented by Cruickshank and Hewett can and are being adapted for use in regular classrooms to assist the learning of children with mild to moderate handicaps. Some educational models provide a resource room or crisis room where the student can receive special help for a portion of the school day. The student remains in the regular classroom the rest of the time. Other hyperactive children can be taught in the regular classroom when the teacher is given support in the form of materials and techniques from an itinerant teacher. Through inservice training, classroom teachers can learn to utilize many of the important instructional techniques without supportive services.

There is a national movement to provide special services based on behavioral descriptions of the child's characteristics rather than traditional categories. These new educational management models (Deno, 1973) attempt to provide a range of educational opportunities for all handicapped children. The goal is to keep the children in the regular classroom whenever possible. The term *mainstreaming* is sometimes used in reference to these new models.

To cite only one example, the *engineered classroom model* described above was developed in the Santa Monica Unified School District. This same school district later developed an alternative program which was called the Madison School Plan (Taylor and Soloway, 1973 and Hewett and Farness, 1974). Children were assigned to various educational services according to their individual readiness to participate in regular class activities. Four levels of competence were delineated—preacademic competence, academic competence, setting competence and reward competence. A special placement inventory was developed to determine the educational placement. The continuum of services ranged from special class placement to consultive services in the regular classroom.

The new instructional alternatives reported by Deno (1973) relate primarily to organizational plans. For the most part, teaching methods and materials of earlier special educational models were adopted or adapted by the innovators. Whether new or old, the common thread of structure runs through all of the literature related to teaching hyperactive or distractible children.

STRUCTURED EDUCATIONAL PLANNING

What is meant by the term *structure* in an educational setting? The word is used repeatedly but seldom defined. Nall (1967) compared structuring the life of a child to that of structuring a house. "If you build a house, you end with a structure. It has limits. It is the same each time you see it (p. 439)." The structured life of a child is based on a plan that is dependable. A structured learning experience involves a plan, a schedule, control and defined limits. Hewett (1968) defined structure as "the 'strings' the teacher attaches to assigned tasks which determine whether or not the rewards present in the classroom will be made available to the child (p. 257)." In other words, according to Hewett, structure determines the what, when, where and how well of an educational plan.

For this discussion the use of structure is divided into five subgroups—structured environment, structured time, structured physical activity, structured rewards and structured tasks. All are important in the formulation of an educational management plan for a hyperactive child.

Structured Environment

Examples of the use of a structured environment in a special class setting were described in the summaries of the Strauss-Lehtinen-Cruickshank and the engineered classroom models. In both examples, the physical plan of the classroom was an important component of the total educational plan.

The structured environment should be based on careful consideration of elements such as room size, desk arrangement, type and size of desks, and control of extraneous environmental stimuli. Many of the structured elements can be employed in regular classrooms when teachers are flexible enough to permit manipulation of the furniture in their classrooms.

‹ A study carrel can be placed in the classroom. When children with learning or behavior problems need to be removed from the distracting elements of the environment, it can be used just as it was advocated in the engineered classroom model. When both teacher and student understand the intention of its use and guidelines are firmly established, the study carrel can be effective in the regular classroom as well as special classrooms.

Teachers should be cautious to use study carrels as aids for learning and not for punishment. It is tempting to the classroom teacher to place the student in a study carrel only when he/she is acting out or disturbing other students in the classroom. This should not be done. Whenever a student has difficulty producing work in a group situation, he should be asked to use the quiet surroundings of the *office*.

Teacher control of the carrel's use is imperative. Some teachers devise a check-in, check-out system to track its use. It is also important to require the student to work while in the office. It should not be a place for the student to avoid his work without being noticed. It is sometimes helpful to set reasonable time limits for successful completion of work in the study carrel.

Study carrels can be purchased from commercial agencies, but they can also be easily made by the teacher. A large cardboard packing box can be cut to fit the need or, for more permanent use, plywood can be used to build the three-sided unit. A regular school desk and chair is placed inside the carrel. An adaptation of the study carrel has been utilized in some classrooms. A three-sided cardboard unit approximately eighteen inches high is available to be placed atop the student's desk when a need to remove visual distractions is apparent.

There is limited research data to support the value of study carrels. They appear to increase attending behavior (Shores and Haubrich, 1969) and, to some extent, performance in arithmetic and quantity of reading assignments completed (Gorton, 1972 and Jenkins, Gorrafa, and Griffiths, 1972). Conversely, the value of study carrels has been questioned by Rost and Charles (1967).

Since sufficient data is not available to dictate their use in all cases, it is a matter of practical experience that prompts many teachers to continue their use for hyperactive and distractible children.

, The placement of the hyperactive child's desk in a classroom is critical. It should not be near distracting areas such as windows and doors, and should be near the area of the room where relevant auditory and visual cues are usually presented. This area is often toward the front of the room.

Hyperactive and distractible children have difficulty man-, aging instructional tools such as pencils, crayons or paper. These distractors are a common source of conflict between teacher and child and between the hyperactive child and his peers. In a structured classroom these tools should be kept in an area separate from the student's desk. The teacher can give the child only those items needed for a particular task. The extra effort on the part of a teacher will be well justified by the number of conflicting situations avoided.

Workbooks commonly kept inside the student's desk should not be placed in the desk of a hyperactive child. It is best to give the child one work page at a time or a packet containing only the day's work. In some cases the work packet can be broken into two parts, one for the morning and one for the afternoon. Preparation of these packets takes advanced planning and time. The preparation provides an excellent opportunity to utilize volunteer help or other students in the classroom. Lehtinen (1948) asked the hyperactive children in her classroom to help prepare their own materials for independent work. They removed visual distractions such as pictures or cut-up work pages and arranged them in simpler formats. Asking children to construct these work pages was seen as an instructional task rather than busy work since the children gained experience in cutting, pasting, measuring, following directions, etc. Obviously this project would take organizational time of the teacher, but it is an interesting idea to be considered in special or regular educational programs.

, Control of extraneous auditory stimuli is another important element of a structured environment. While this element is easily controlled in special classrooms, it is more difficult to control in regular classrooms. One approach to meeting this challenge is to provide the hyperactive child a headset or sound muffler he can^d use during study periods. This technique is not unique to teaching hyperactive children. Even college students find headsets helpful when they try to study in noisy dormatories.

What happens to the hyperactive child in an open classroom? The modern concept of open classroom teaching in which large groups of students are taught by teams of teachers in spacious and busy environments would appear to spell disaster for hyperactive children. It is true that some hyperactive children have difficulty functioning in such an environmental setting, but others cope quite well. In fact, since these classrooms are often well equipped to meet individual needs through a variety of programming structures, they have potential to provide the type of structure described by Hewett better than many special classrooms or regular self-contained classrooms. While the open classroom appears to be the antithesis of a structured environment, the question is really one of degree and type of structure. Discovery of ways to bring together the open classroom structure and the contingency management structure for benefit of hyperactive children may be a fruitful direction for future research. A teacher training package that deals with this issue is Volkmor, C., Langstaff, A., and Higgins, M., *Structuring the Classroom for Success.*

Structured Time

‹ Another use of structure for hyperactive children is the structuring of time. A common complaint by parents and teachers alike is "he/she doesn't complete his/her work on *time."* Teachers frequently assign independent work only to find the hyperactive child does not get beyond the first two or three problems. A teacher might assign a report on Monday asking for completion by Friday. The hyperactive child might work on the assignment on Monday and never again, or he/she might wait until Friday to begin. Such students are labeled lazy, irresponsible, forgetful, sloppy or other useless terms. The teacher who is concerned about helping these children must find ways to structure their time.

In special classroom programs, time is structured through the use of schedules that provide a variety of short work periods. Children with short attention spans are given assignments equal to their limited abilities. It is more difficult to structure time for a child in a regular classroom, but not impossible. For example, in one second grade classroom the teacher prepared a card each day that listed each activity or task that the child was expected to complete and assigned time limits when appropriate. The child was asked to put a check mark beside the item on his/her card when the task or activity was completed. The card was taped to the child's desk since it was easily lost otherwise. This simple technique was helpful to the child who began completing his/her assignments with regularity and remained in his/her seat for longer periods of time without interrupting the teacher.

The hyperactive child can seldom attend to a task for the same length of time as his/her normal peers. This shorter attention span is a source of frustration to the classroom teacher. It is important to give the student work assignments that can be completed within his/her own limitations. This often requires breaking a long assignment into several shorter ones. In upper grades it involves daily assignments rather than weekly assignments. In math it might involve an assignment of three problems rather than six.

Behavioral modification techniques can be helpful in the structure of time. Rewards or reinforcers that follow completion of tasks within a selected time period serve to structure conformity to time. One application of this concept was made by Hewett (1968) in the engineered classroom.

It is not necessary to use tangible reinforcers such as tokens or trinkets. The exchange of one type of time—work time—for another type of time—play time—is often effective. Classroom teachers have always used this type of exchange by depriving the child who did not complete his/her work of a recess period. This reinforcement was in the form of punishment and therefore negative. Modern behaviorists would encourage a positive approach by instructing the child that when his/her work is completed, he/ she will be given play time. In this approach, which is sometimes called contingency management, the child who completes his/her work in a short amount of time is rewarded with a longer play period than the student who uses a longer period of time to complete his/her work. Successful use of this contingency model requires planning to control the reasonable expectations of the work period.

⟩ The hyperactive child is not a good waiter. Waiting in lines, waiting for lunch, waiting for help or waiting for nothing is an intolerable situation for the hyperactive child. During such wait- ⟩ ing periods the teacher faces more behavior problems than any other portion of the school day. The teacher who structures classroom time appropriately will avoid such waiting periods.

⟩ Most hyperactive children rush. They are impulsive or disinhibited according to some definitions. Some educational problems appear to be the result of this impulsive behavior. The structure of time, helping the child to use more time on a selected task, may be beneficial to such students.

In a structured classroom the teacher should be conscious of his/her own use of time. The teacher is an organizer and facilitator of schedules. The amount of time a teacher spends giving instructions should be controlled (Cruickshank, 1968). This logical suggestion is often overlooked by teachers who are eager to make instructions clear. Redundancy of instructions might serve to confuse rather than clarify the issues.

⟩ The importance of structure of time for hyperactive children cannot be overstated. Schedules and routines give the child a feeling of consistency and security.

Structured Physical Activity

⟩ A teacher of a hyperactive child dreads the thought of taking the students to the gymnasium or out on the playground because the hyperactive child in the group will usually return to the classroom ready to tear it apart. "Let him run off his extra energy" is not sound advice for the teacher or parent of a hyperactive child. The overstimulation of physical activity is overwhelming to these children.

For some children with learning problems the only place to experience success is on the playground, but for the hyperactive child with learning problems the playground is often an arena of failure greater than the classroom experience. Poor gross and fine motor coordination are common characteristics among hyperactive children, especially those children whose problems are neurologically-based. These children need physical activity programs designed to meet their individual needs. Motor development should be remediated through a structured physical education program to assure the child success in this important area of learning.

In special classrooms for hyperactive children, physical activity is usually limited to calm stretching-bending exercises in the early phases of the special programs. As the children learn self-control, organized games are included in the plan. When active organized games are planned, explicit instructions should be given before leaving the classroom. Hyperactive children are unable to listen effectively in the highly stimulating environment of the playground.

After physical activities, hyperactive children benefit from a relaxation period. Such a period helps them focus attention on the academic situation to follow. The relaxation period can be as simple as turning down the lights while the children rest their heads on their desks for a few minutes. Structured relaxation activities are described by Cratty and Martin (1969) who used them with hyperactive children. These activities were based on the work of Jacobson (1938).

Limitations of perceptual-motor training programs were cited in the introduction of this chapter. There is a danger that educators will overreact to these warnings and eliminate all physical education programs designed to develop motor ability for children with deficits in this area. Elimination of these programs is not the intent. While motor training programs should not be substitutes for academic programs, and their effectiveness for training skills that will transfer to academic learning has been questioned, they should not be eliminated from the educational plan for hyperactive children. Suggestions for structured physical activities for handicapped children are available in the following works: Barsch, R., *A Movigenic Curriculum;* Barsch, R., *Achieving Perceptual-motor Efficiency;* Barsch, R., *Enriching Perception and Cognition, vol. 2.;* Frostig, M., and Horne, D., *The Frostig Program for the Development of Visual Perception;* Gerhardt, L., *Moving and Knowing: The Young Child Orients Himself in Space;* Getman, G., Kane, E., Halgren, M., and McKee, G, *The Physiology of Readiness, an Action Program for the Development of Perception for Children;* Hammill, D., and Bartel, N., *Teaching Children with Learning and Behavioral Problems.* Kephart, N., *The Slow Learner in the Classroom;* and Lerner, J., *Children with Learning Difficulties.*

Structured Rewards

Teachers have long recognized the powerful effects of rewards in the classroom. Bright learners gain easily their share of classroom rewards such as praise, good grades, positive comments on papers, teacher smiles or pats on the back. Since these consequences are not a natural outcome of the hyperactive child's school experience, the teacher must structure a situation that guarantees rewards for him.

Structured use of rewards is an important component of the engineered classroom and is gaining acceptance in most special education classrooms and some regular classrooms as well. Structured rewards refers to behavior modification techniques or systematic application of behavioral principles. A detailed discussion of behavior modification techniques is presented in the chapter by Rieth.

Structured Tasks

Structure of instructional tasks is probably the most important consideration in teaching hyperactive children. The term *structure* in this context refers to the systematic planning of instructional tasks. While teachers may not be able to control the total educational program, the selection and implementation of instructional tasks is the teacher's primary responsibility.

Some hyperactive children do *not* appear to have associated learning problems. These children should profit from normal instructional tasks of the regular classroom. Other hyperactive children may be intellectually gifted. In fact, it may be boredom that causes these children to exhibit hyperactive behavior. The gifted child should be provided instructional tasks that are challenging and intellectually stimulating. For most hyperactive children, learning performance is inconsistent and below the level expected for their ages and mental abilities. To reverse this failure pattern, carefully structured and individualized instructional tasks are necessary.

The teacher can attempt to fit the child to the task or he/she can fit the task to the child. For example, the teacher can set goals to increase the attending behavior of the child, thereby permitting completion of a task assigned to his/her normal peers, or, given the knowledge that the child has a short attention span, the assignment can be shortened to be compatible with the child's attention span. In many instances, attempts to fit the child to the task have not been successful. The most promising approach is to fit the task to the child. The alternative chosen depends on the situation. The best solution might be an interaction of both approaches.

In either approach, the structure of the instructional task involves careful analysis of two aspects—the nature of the child and the nature of the task. The instructional planning should involve the following steps leading to an individualized program for each child:

1. Determine the nature of the child.

2. Select instructional priorities.

3. Determine the nature of the task.

4. Choose the method most suitable for the child.

5. Adopt or adapt materials to fit the child's need.

Instructional planning is an ongoing process based on daily evaluation of student response and feedback.

Determine the Nature of the Child

To arrange instructional tasks that will meet the needs of an individual student it is necessary first to know as much as possible about his/her psychological and academic strengths and weaknesses. This information is obtained through a systematic diagnostic process. Diagnosis can be either formal or informal. In most instances the formal diagnosis is based on a clinical-medical model while informal diagnosis is compatible with behavioral models. The two approaches are not discrete, and many diagnosticians combine parts of both in their evaluations.

Formal diagnosis involves the use of standardized instruments to compare the student's ability to that of a normative group. This level of diagnosis usually identifies general areas of strength and weakness. The diagnosis should utilize individual assessment measures in a controlled testing environment. Formal diagnostic batteries can assess areas such as intelligence, language development, perceptual skills, motor skills, affective development or academic areas such as reading, arithmetic, handwriting or spelling.

In most instances the evaluator must have special training to administer and interpret the tests. Sometimes a single diagnostician such as a school psychologist will perform the total diagnostic function. In other situations a multidisciplinary team will evaluate the child, each team member viewing the child from his/her own disciplinary background. It is necessary for the diagnostic team to confer and recommend a remedial plan based on the results of their findings. The educational specialist or teacher is responsible for implementing the instructional plan while other team members attend to the child's needs in other ways.

For purposes of structuring instructional tasks, data from academic skill tests are the most useful. For example, it is more helpful to the teacher to know that the student has a poor sight vocabulary than it is to know his/her IQ is 95. At best, formal diagnostic instruments can only sample important skill areas. Many diagnostic instruments provide little more than an estimate of achievement levels. Perhaps the greatest value of formal measures is to provide a cross-section sampling to identify areas for further probing through informal assessment procedures.

From an educational point of view, the diagnosis is sterile if change in the educational program does not evolve from the findings. If the diagnostic report is too technical or nondirective the individual responsible for selecting or structuring the educational tasks for the child, such as the classroom teacher, will not benefit from the diagnostic efforts. It is the responsibility of the diagnostician or diagnostic team to interpret and define the results of the evaluation in educationally-relevant terms if changes in the instructional program are expected.

Informal diagnosis involves the use of teacher-made criterion measures to probe for minute and precise areas of instructional need. For example, formal measures may indicate the student does not know phonic analysis. Through informal assessment, however, the teacher may determine the student does not know initial blends, diagraphs and unglided vowels. Probing further, the teacher may discover the student knows the blends bl, dr, cr and fl, but all other blends are unknown. This type of information yields specific data to formulate instructional tasks. Good teachers have always used informal measures of diagnosis, but for children with learning problems the teacher must use them systematically.

Some teachers are not able to structure an informal diagnostic procedure because they do not have sufficient knowledge of the content area to perform a task analysis that will delineate the important subskills. It is impossible to informally diagnose reading problems, for example, if the evaluator does not know the subskills of reading and have a comprehensive understanding of the reading process. Commercially produced, criterion-referenced tests may be useful as a transition stage between formal and informal testing procedures. The teacher may also utilize a scope and sequence chart to determine the subskills that should be measured.

The diagnostic process is not a simple matter. Error is common whether testing is formal or informal. Formal tests do not always measure the precise skills claimed for them. Likewise, teachers do not always construct tests that measure the exact behavior they wish to assess. For example, a teacher might want to know if the student can read initial consonant sounds. To measure the skill, the teacher pronounces a word and asks the student to write the beginning letter. Such a task does not measure ability to read, although it does measure the student's ability to write initial consonants. Admittedly, the writing task is related to the reading task—for most children the correlation between the two is high. For children with learning problems the teacher can never assume that ability to write assures ability to read. Nor can it be assumed that failure to write assures failure to read. To assess reading skill, the student must be asked to read.

Diagnosis is never an end in itself but the beginning of an ongoing process in diagnostic teaching. Diagnostic data usually reveal many areas in need of remediation or special planning. The diagnostic evaluation can be used as an initial step for establishing priorities for intervention.

References describing formal and informal diagnosis of academic skills include Bond, G., and Tinker, M., *Reading Difficulties: Their Diagnosis and Correction, 2nd ed.;* Della-Piana, G., *Reading Diagnosis and Prescription;* Guszak, F., *Diagnostic Reading Instruction in the Elementary School;* Hammill, D., and Bartel, N., *Teaching Children With Learning and Behavior Problems;* Harris, A., *How to Increase Reading Ability, 5th ed.,* Johnson, D., and Myklebust, H., *Learning Disabilities: Educational Principles and Practices;* Lerner, J., *Children With Learning Disabilities;* Mann, P., and Suiter, P., *Handbook in Diagnostic Teaching: A Learning Disabilities Approach;* and Otto, W., McMenemy, R., and Smith, R., *Corrective and Remedial Teaching, 2nd ed.*

Select Instructional Priorities

The purpose of diagnosis is to systematically determine areas of strength and weakness as a means of selecting instructional goals for the individual student. For most students with learning problems the diagnostic profile will provide clues that lead to identification of many important learning goals. It is impossible to teach everything at one time, and the teacher must select priorities for long-term and short-term goals. The short-term goals should be accomplished during a single teaching session and should be sequential steps leading to completion of broader long-term goals.

The process of selecting priorities is somewhat arbitrary and based on the teacher's knowledge of the child and theoretical bias. Some educators believe it is important to identify priorities within a developmental framework, beginning with preacademic skills and progressing to higher cognitive levels in a sequential manner. Other teachers limit priorities to academic-level tasks while another group remediates perceptual and language processes concurrently with academic skills.

All educators agree the most important consideration in selection of priorities is to provide a large measure of success. The child who has experienced repeated failure in school needs success to reassure him that academic learning is possible for him. Cruickshank (1967) stated it this way, "It is essential, then, for the teacher to carefully assess the skills of the child in all aspects of his learning and to find a level of competence so primitive that success is possible, not on a chance basis, but continuously. On this primitive level then, other learnings are based (p. 56)."

Success is loosely defined as the level of performance that has almost no error. To assure success, new concepts and skills are planned and introduced at a slow and carefully sequenced pace. The teacher might arbitrarily select 95 percent to 99 percent accuracy as an estimate of success. For children with serious learning difficulties it is not always possible to provide success in academic skill tasks. It might be necessary to select preacademic level tasks for these children, even if the student is beyond the primary grade level in age.

The instructional priorities should be stated in behavioral terms. These objectives should be observable and measureable. According to Mager (1962) an instructional objective should

1. Identify a terminal behavior by name; you can specify the kind of behavior that will be accepted as evidence that the learner has achieved the objective.
2. Try to define the desired behavior further by describing the important conditions under which the behavior will be expected to occur.
3. Specify the criteria of acceptable performance by describing how well the performer must perform to be considered acceptable (p. 12).

Statements of instructional objectives provide an important foundation for further educational planning.

Determine the Nature of the Task

After the teacher has determined what to teach, the task must be broken into a sequence of small steps. The process of determining these steps is usually called task analysis. Task analysis requires the teacher to think logically about how the task can be learned. The teacher can ask "What are the components of the task and what is the logical order for them?" Most commercially prepared instructional materials do not break the task into small enough steps for children with learning problems to progress with success. The teacher must add the interim steps if commercially prepared materials are used. In addition, knowledge of the child's unique characteristics can necessitate modifications of a sequence typically used. For example, if the student has serious auditory problems the teacher might choose to delay introduction of certain phonic elements in reading and spelling or, if they are introduced, might add more steps at the perceptual level.

The process of task analysis is not an easy, natural function of teaching. The teacher's knowledge of the content area, ability to think logically and understanding of learning theory are critical elements for successful completion of task analysis. It would be ludicrous for this writer to attempt a task analysis of replacing a TV tube, but task analysis of writing the letter "A" is a possibility. The former content is not familiar to the writer while the latter is. In this example the ability to think logically had nothing to do with success in task analysis. To use task analysis effectively, then, teachers need thorough training in the content area they will attempt to teach along with an understanding of the proce ses of teaching and learning.

With task analysis the teacher must not only determine the possible subskills but should consider what Popham and Baker (1970) call "instructional economy"—that is, "it is possible to identify more behaviors as enroute than are necessary to the efficient attainment of the objective." The number of steps selected for an individual child is determined by knowledge of his/her level of achievement, learning rate, age, interests and other related factors. Siegel (1972) lists the following criteria for task analysis:

1. The aim of the sequence should be well-defined and somewhat limited rather than general. . .
2. The behavioral objective must be an observable one. . .
3. The number of steps must not be so large as to overwhelm the teacher; yet the gaps must be sufficiently narrow to allow the teacher to gain a footing and to see how to proceed from step to step. . .
4. Generally, the increasing difficulty of each step should be visible and able to pass the test of face validity. . .
5. Some instructions to the teacher are necessary, yet the specific methodology should not be spelled out. . .
6. General areas of difficulty should be anticipated and the suggested coping strategies incorporated into the sequence. . .
7. In attempting to design a sequence for a specific aim, the teacher must not feel that there is only one set of steps which will satisfy the requirements of the task. . .
8. Great care should be taken with the layout itself, lest the reader find it overwhelming, similar to the imponderables found in the printed instructions in some of the commercial assembly kits. . . (pp. 89-95).

The sequence of activities should be analyzed to determine ways to enhance meaning. If each new step is connected with a previous experience, the learning task will be easier. Special consideration should also be given to position of difficult items in a sequence. It is a well-established psychological principle that the beginning and ending of a sequence is learned more rapidly than the items positioned just past the middle. In consideration of this important principle, Hunter (1969) cites five practical suggestions for consideration in arranging the instructional sequence. Since hyperactive children often have difficulties in retaining sequential information, these suggestions are especially useful to the teacher of hyperactive children.

The first suggestion advanced by Hunter (1969) relates to rearranging the sequence if it is possible. The position of the just-past-the-middle item can be changed so it occurs in the first or last position. Perhaps the most meaningful element could be placed in the middle position since it is easiest to learn. In spelling, for example, the shortest or phonetically-regular words could hold the middle position of the sequence since they are easiest to learn. Many other variations of this concept can be applied, depending on the nature of the sequence to be learned.

If the order of the sequence cannot be changed, a second approach suggested by Hunter (1969 p. 44) is to " (1) establish the order of the sequence, (2) pull out the material occupying the just-past-the-middle position, (3) work on it separately and (4) then replace it in the sequence." For example, when learning to spell a multisyllable word, the total word can be studied initially, then the medial syllable can be pulled out for separate analysis and study and, finally, the total word can be reviewed and rehearsed.

The third suggestion is use of a chaining technique. With this approach, the last portion of the sequence is taught first. The remainder of the sequence is taught in order but in a reverse manner. For example, when teaching a child to tie his shoes, the teacher completes all steps except the final one which is completed by the student after demonstration. In the next lesson, the student completes the last two steps and so on. The technique can be used in game-like activities where the teacher spells a word, omitting the final letter which is supplied by the students, then spells the word again omitting the last two letters for the children to supply, etc. In this way, the last association learned is the first task the student must perform in the total sequence. Chaining is not often used in school learning tasks but should be considered as an alternative for students with serious learning problems in sequential memory.

As a fourth alternative, the sequence can be learned in the usual manner and the middle portion can then be reviewed at the end of the lesson; finally, the learning task can be broken into smaller units to avoid interference of learning the middle portion. This latter alternative is the most commonly recommended procedure for teaching children with learning problems, but the teacher of hyperactive children should also consider the other suggestions when planning an instructional sequence for individual students.

The selection of an instructional sequence, then, is a critical component of structuring tasks. It is technical and requires a great deal of sophistication on the part of the teacher. In many instances the teacher will be able to use commercially prepared instructional materials to assist her in developing the sequence, but overdependence on materials might repeat a pattern of inappropriate teaching.

Choose the Method Most Suitable for the Child

Selection of an instructional sequence has nothing to do with the teaching method. Most instructional sequences can be taught through a variety of methods. The most appropriate method is determined by an understanding of the student's abilities, learning style, preferences, biases, affective needs, etc. The diagnostic information forms a basis for this knowledge of the student's characteristics.

If the student appears to learn best when information is presented visually, then the method can stress visual input. If the student has difficulty writing, the method can omit written responses. If the student is an adolescent who needs to learn beginning reading skills, the method can appeal to his mature interest rather than the activities typically used for beginning reading. The variety of considerations for selection of method is beyond the scope of this discussion. A few special methods are described because they appear to have relevance for hyperactive students. They do not represent an exhaustive exploration of the topic.

Several special reading methods have been effectively utilized with some hyperactive children. These methods involve techniques that appear to have the effect of focussing the student's attention on the relevant stimuli in the reading process. For example, one aspect of the Fernald Approach (Fernald, 1943) requires the student to study unknown words as whole words utilizing a combination of visual, auditory, kinesthetic and tactile sensory input. A word is written with crayon on a card and the student traces the word with his/her finger as he sees it and pronounces it. Then he attempts to write the word from memory and checks it for accuracy. Words are taught for mastery, and the amount of stimulus required for learning new words is gradually reduced.

Another reading program that is highly structured and multisensory was developed by Gillingham and Stillman (1966). This reading, spelling and writing program differs from the Fernald approach in that the student learns word parts first and then synthesizes them into whole words, sentences and stories. Again, mastery learning is emphasized and associations are reinforced through multisensory stimulus and response.

Two other remedial methods may be effective for improving accuracy and fluency in reading but are not total reading programs. They should be considered for use in the reading programs of older hyperactive children who have mastered the basic reading skills but persist in oral reading fluency errors during connected reading, a behavior common among impulsive students (Kagan, 1965). The first is called the *neurological impress method* (Heckelman, 1969) and the second, *pencil facilitation* (Ansara, 1972).

With the neurological impress method, the student and teacher read in unison as the student slides his/her finger along the line of print. It is important to syncronize the moving finger with the flow of words. Student errors are ignored as the teacher reads the words correctly. Each reading session lasts about fifteen minutes daily.

The pencil facilitation technique utilizes the pencil during oral reading and later during silent reading. Initially, the first letter of each word is traced as it is pronounced. When accuracy has improved, the first letter is simply underlined rather than traced. At the next stage the student merely runs the pencil under each line without lifting it. Ansara (1972) believes the penciling technique helps to maintain focus and to overcome rotations, regression, transpositions, insertions, substitutions and omissions in reading.

These remedial approaches may be effective because they have the effect of forcing the student to slow down or mediate responses. The use of verbal inhibitory commands may also be beneficial for this purpose. Teachers should try various approaches to help the student reflect before responding and to interfere with the impulsivity of his/her response.

The structure of the instructional method should provide the student with practice and immediate feedback. One approach for structuring these elements is the use of charts. Classroom teachers have always used charts to record performance of students in the classroom, but behavioral scientists have encouraged the use of charts to systematically record individual student performance. The charts serve as feedback and pinpoint the need for reteaching, practice or drill. An experimental method using charts for instructional purposes is known as "precision teaching" (Haring, 1973; Haring, 1974; and Haring and Phillips, 1972). When this method is used, a behavioral goal is first identified. Systematic sampling and recording of performance on charts provide an ongoing measure and record of the progress toward reaching the goal. The teaching methods utilized in the instructional task can be modified or changed when the data indicate that progress is not evident. Measurements are taken daily or at least in short time intervals to provide constant feedback to both teacher and child.

Although research data is not available to support or reject the efficacy of precision teaching for hyperactive children, there is some evidence that the highly structured nature of the process is beneficial to these students. Critics of the technique pinpoint as limitations the expenditure of time and the mechanistic nature of the process. The technique is not easy to use without special training (Haring, 1973). Teachers desiring to use the approach should study it carefully before beginning.

Other suggestions for useful methods of teaching hyperactive children are presented by Connor, J., *Classroom Activities for Helping Hyperactive Children;* Cruickshank, W., Bentzen, F., Ratzburg, F., and Tannhauser, M., *A Teaching Method for Brain-injured and Hyperactive Children;* Hammill, D., and Bartel, N., *Teaching Children with Learning and Behavior Problems;* Haring, N., and Phillips, E., *Educating Emotionally Disturbed Children;* Harris, A., *How to Increase Reading Ability, 5th ed.;* Hewett, F., *The Emotionally Disturbed Child in the Classroom;* Johnson, D., and Myklebust, H., *Learning Disabilities: Educational Principles and Practices;* Lerner, J., *Children With Learning Disabilities;* Myers, P., and Hammill, D., *Methods for Learning Disorders;* Otto, W., McMenemy, R., and Smith, R., *Corrective and Remedial Teaching, 2nd ed.;* and Wallace, G., and Kauffman, J., *Teaching Children With Learning Problems.*

Adopt or Adapt Materials to Fit the Child's Need

After decisions have been made to determine what to teach, the order for teaching it and how to teach it, the teacher must decide what to use to teach it. This requires a selection, adaptation or development of instructional materials.

During the past decade a variety of instructional materials have been produced and disseminated on the commercial market. Many of these materials were designed specifically for students with learning problems. They can readily be adopted for use with some hyperactive children. To adopt instructional materials for children with learning and behavioral problems, the teacher should ask questions such as those listed in the *Checklist to Adopt/Adapt Instructional Materials* presented in Figure 1.

Frequently it is necessary for the teacher to adapt portions of the materials for effective use. Adaptations might involve changing the mode of input from visual to auditory, dividing a lesson into several shorter parts, rearranging the spacing or highlighting important cues.

Strauss and Lehtinen (1947) and Cruickshank (1961) believed instructional materials should be adapted to remove unnecessary distractions and to highlight relevant cues. Pictures were removed from the instructional materials. Workbook pages

CHECKLIST TO ADOPT/ADAPT INSTRUCTIONAL MATERIALS

	YES	NO	ADAPTATION
CONTENT EVALUATION:			
Is it consistent with instructional goals?			
Will it appeal to the interest of the student?			
Is the sequence appropriate for the student?			
Is the readability level appropriate?			
Are lessons short enough to fit the attention span of the student?			
Are there opportunities for practice and feedback?			
Are evaluation components included?			
Are directions clearly stated?			
Will the mode of input/output allow the student to use his strength?			
FORMAT EVALUATION			
Is it durably constructed?			
Is it attractive enough to solicit interest without overstimulation?			
Are visual distractions minimal?			
Is spacing of content adequate?			
Does color call attention to important cues?			
Is the print size large enough for this student?			
Are all components easy to manipulate?			
Are all necessary materials included?			
Is special equipment included?			
Are audio components clearly recorded and free from distractions?			
Is the speaking rate appropriate?			
Can it be used in the proposed organizational structure-group, individual, etc.?			

Figure 4-1.

were cut up, leaving only the relevant stimuli. Cruickshank (1961 p. 165) stated,

> The teacher tries to provide motor activity which engages the child directly in his task and which fixes his attention on the process involved. She tries to create materials that are self-tutoring, so that the child is helped to become independent of the teacher. She designs materials that are free of unnecessary detail, that do not distract the child, and that enable him to focus his attention on the task at hand. For example, she uses only simple forms. The child is to think of color or form and is not to be distracted by cats, trees, or rabbits.

Color was used in a variety of creative ways by these early researchers. For example, the various strokes in writing were presented in different colors. Special writing paper with top and bottom lines in contrasting colors was used. Different number patterns were presented in different colors, gradually removing the color cue in the task. In writing numeral combinations, a different color was used for each number, with the function sign in yet another color. This technique was used during the initial phases of instruction, again with a gradual removal of the color cue after the association was learned. Creative teachers can use color in many other ways to enhance instruction for children with learning problems. It usually involves minimal adaptation of materials by simply tracing over letters with colored ink.

In a recent study of the value of color cues in paired-associate learning, Allington (1975) pointed out the hazard of using color cues which can result in the student forming associations with the color rather than the primary stimulus, i.e. letter shapes. He concluded that when a single color hue is used, this problem is minimized, and when the colors are gradually vanished, i.e. a form of fading or reducing the area of color rather than the intensity of saturation, effectiveness was further increased.

Sometimes media can be helpful to structure the instructional task of the hyperactive child. Educational technology has only scratched the surface of the potential of a variety of media in education. Hyperactive children may benefit from the use of audio cassettes with headsets rather than classroom lecture since extraneous auditory stimuli can be reduced.

Hyperactive students who have visual-motor difficulties can use the tape recorder as a substitute for written responses. These same students might benefit from the use of a typewriter to compensate for the poor handwriting they have acquired. Teachers are discovering daily other exciting opportunities to help students through the use of media.

When appropriate instructional materials are not available, the teacher will find it necessary to create materials. The teacher should be certain that these materials are clearly written, free of distractions and have items spaced farther apart than is usual. If they are duplicated, he/she should be certain the copy is dark and easily read.

Teachers should always remember that instructional materials are only a means to an end. The most beautifully mediated materials are useless if the content and sequence is not relevant for the individual student.

The implementation of the structured task is the ultimate goal for the teacher. The synthesis of all elements of structure should result in a successful learning experience for the student. If it does not, the teacher must evaluate the results and modify future plans based on the student's performance. Additionally, the student should be given immediate feedback to allow him/her to modify his/her own behavior.

The use of structure in the educational management of hyperactive children is widely accepted. The precise nature or degree of structure is debated, and the final decision must be based on the needs of each individual child, the resources available and the teacher's ability to provide structure. Many aspects of structure are applicable to all children with learning and behavior problems whether hyperactivity is a behavioral characteristic or not. When other forms of behavioral control such as the use of medication are effective, the direct use of structure in the educational plan can be minimized. Responsibility for structuring the instructional task remains the most important element in the educational management of all children, including hyperactive children.

SUMMARY

It is clear that no single educational program or strategy is suitable for all hyperactive children. Within the general class of hyperactive children there are many individuals. The educational management of each individual must be determined by a thorough understanding of his/her strengths and weaknesses—his social, emotional, physical and cognitive needs. The type of educational plan advocated is often based on the relationship perceived between hyperactivity and the learning problem. Keogh (1971) hypothesized at least three different reasons for school learning problems among hyperactive children. Each hypothesis has implications for different educational interventions.

The educational management of hyperactive children in the United States has been strongly influenced by special class models. Two examples were presented in this chapter. The Strauss-Lehtinen-Cruickshank model grew out of clinical-medical research with brain-damaged subjects. Hyperactivity and distractibility, along with perceptual and conceptual disorders, were associated with brain damage in the early work of Strauss and Lehtinen. Cruickshank identified behavioral symptoms among children who did not have a clinical diagnosis of brain damage and applied the teaching techniques of Strauss and Lehtinen to hyperactive children with or without brain damage. The primary consideration of the Strauss-Lehtinen-Cruickshank model involves reduction of unessential environmental stimuli, reduction of environmental space, a highly structured daily program, and an increased stimulus value in the instructional materials.

The model described by Hewett (1968) has many similarities to the Strauss-Lehtinen-Cruickshank model, but it stresses the use of behavioral modification techniques. The hyperactive children of concern to Hewett were called emotionally disturbed without regard for physical etiology such as brain damage. Hewett did not adhere to the extreme approach of removing unessential environmental stimuli, but he advocated a highly structured daily schedule with instructional tasks and rewards equally structured. Both experimental models report positive though somewhat tentative results in control of behavior and learning in their subjects. Since most educators are *eclectic* in their application of research, parts of both approaches are utilized in many special education classrooms throughout the United States.

The application of structure in the educational management of hyperactive children is the most significant element of both models. It is the most universally accepted concept relative to the teaching of hyperactive children. Structure relates to the plan, organization or control of all components of the educational program. Structure of at least five elements should be considered— structured environment, structured time, structured physical activity, structured rewards and structured tasks. Each of these elements of structure has been discussed in this chapter. Each can be applied in varying degrees depending upon the need of the child and the resources available to the teacher.

Whether or not the educational structure should be provided in a special setting, in the regular classroom or in a modified plan such as in a resource room is an issue that remains to be resolved. As late as 1967 Cruickshank insisted that a special class was essential for hyperactive children. He stated,

> Recommendation for special class placement is made by one who is known to feel that the goal of all special education is the integration of the child into the normal educational program insofar as possible and as quickly as possible. These children present too many unique differences to permit their easy, convenient or appropriate retention in the regular grade. Special facilities are required if they are ultimately to reassume a place in the normal educational stream (p. 57).

Decisions regarding educational placement must necessarily be a matter of judgment based on a thorough understanding of each individual. Schools must make available a continuum of services, allowing flexibility in decisions of educational placement. A variety of instructional models and alternatives was reported by Deno (1973). These experimental programs brought out the need for involvement of the total educational community in planning for handicapped children. It is not reasonable to remove the student from the mainstream of education without a system for reintegrating him back into the stream when sufficient improvement is made. This position has grown out of educational research and experience in which removal of handicapped children from their normal peers has resulted in a difficult transition back into the normal social structure.

The *mainstreaming* concept will be useful for hyperactive children only if (1) supportive human and material resources are provided for the classroom teacher and (2) the teacher is taught methods for structuring the educational program in the classroom. These processes will require changes in preservice and in-service education. Classroom teachers today are providing more individualized instruction, more application of contingency management and other behavior modification techniques, and more humanistic acceptance of individual differences than traditional classrooms permitted, but there remains a need for improved skills to manage hyperactive children effectively. This writer was involved in in-service education of more than 400 regular classroom teachers throughout the state of Kansas during the 1974-1975 school year. It was observed that the problems of managing hyperactive and aggressive children in the classroom were a high priority need identified by these teachers.

Educational management of hyperactive children is probably the most difficult of all areas of exceptionality. The problems are both behavioral and cognitive. Such children are truly multiply handicapped. They challenge educators to apply the most precise techniques available to the profession. Hyperactive children with profound disabilities will always need the services of special classes and teachers who are artists in applying structure to the teaching situation. Many hyperactive children will be successful in one of several alternative models that provide special help for only part of the school day, but others will function comfortably in the regular classroom if the teacher is given supportive resources.

While educators and other professionals debate the most appropriate intervention strategy for these children, researchers continue to discover new methods and techniques for helping them. Until such time as new discoveries are made, one principle remains for the teacher of hyperactive children—these children *can* learn if the educational program provides structure that includes consistency, control, concern and commitment.

REFERENCES

Abeson, A., and Blacklow, J.: *Environmental Design: New Relevance For Special Education.* Arlington, Council for Exceptional Children, 1971.

Allen, K., Henke, L., Baer, D., and Reynolds, N.: Control of hyperactivity by social reinforcement of attending behavior. *J Ed Psychol, 58*:231-37, 1967.

Allington, R.: An evaluation of the use of color cues to focus attention in discrimination and paired-associate learning. *Reading Res O, 10*(2):244-247, 1974-75.

Ansara, A.: Language therapy to salvage the college potential of dyslexic adolescents. *Bull Orton Soc, 22*:123-139, 1972.

Barsch, R.: *A Movigenic Curriculum.* Madison, State Dept. Of Public Instruction, Bureau for the Handicapped, 1965.

Barsch, R.: *Achieving Perceptual-motor Efficiency.* Seattle, Spec Child, 1967.

Barsch, R.: *Enriching Perception and Cognition,* Seattle, Spec Child, vol. 2, 1968.

Bond, G., and Tinker, M.: *Reading Difficulties: Their Diagnosis and Correction, 2nd ed.* New York, Appleton, 1967.

Connor, J.: *Classroom Activities for Helping Hyperactive Children.* New York, Center for Applied Research in Education, 1974.

Cratty, B., and Martin, M.: *Perceptual-motor Efficiency in Children.* Philadelphia, Lea & Feibiger, 1969.

Cruickshank, W.: Hyperactive children: Their needs and curriculum. In Knoblock, P., and Johnson, J. (Eds.): *The Teaching-Learning Process in Educating Emotially Disturbed Children,* Syracuse, University Pr, 13210, 1967.

Cruickshank, W., Bentzen, F., Ratzburg, F., and Tannhauser, M.: *A Teaching Method for Brain-injured and Hyperactive Children.* Syracuse, Syracuse U Pr, 1961.

Delacato, C.: *The Treatment and Prevention of Reading Problems: The Neurological Approach.* Springfield, Thomas, 1959.

Della-Piana, G.: *Reading Diagnosis and Prescription.* New York, HR & W, 1968.

Deno, E.: *Instructional Alternatives for Exceptional Children.* Arlington, Council for Exceptional Children, 1973.

Fernald, G.: *Remedial Techniques in Basic School Subjects.* New York, McGraw, 1943.

Frostig, M., and Horne, D.: *The Frostig Program for the Development of Visual Perception.* Chicago, Follett, 1964.

Gerhardt, L.: *Moving and Knowing: The Young Child Orients Himself in Space.* Englewood Cliffs, P-H, 1973.

Getman, G., Kane, E., Halgren, M., and McKee, G.: *The Physiology of Readiness, an Action Program for the Development of Perception for Children.* Minneapolis, Programs to Accelerate Success, 1964.

Gillingham, A., and Stillman, B.: *Remedial Training for Children With Specific Difficulty in Reading, Spelling, and Penmanship,* 7th ed. Cambridge, Ed Pub Serv, 1966.

Gorton, C.: The effects of various classroom environments on performance of a mental task by mentally retarded and normal children. *Education and Training of the Mentally Retarded, 7:*32-38, 1972.

Guszak, F.: *Diagnostic Reading Instruction in the Elementary School.* New York, Har Row, 1972.

Hallahan, D., and Cruickshank, W.: *Psychoeducational Foundations of Learning Disabilities.* Englewood Cliffs, P-H, 1973.

Hammill, D., and Bartel, N.: *Teaching Children With Learning and Behavior Problems.* Boston, Allyn, 1975.

Haring, N.: *Behavior of Exceptional Children: An Introduction to Special Education.* Columbus, Merrill, 1974.

Haring, H., and Phillips, E.: *Analysis and Modification of Classroom Behavior.* Englewood Cliffs, P-H, 1972.

Haring, N., and Phillips, E.: *Educating Emotionally Disturbed Children.* New York, McGraw, 1962.

Haring, N., and Whelan, R. (Ed.): *The Learning Environment: Relationship to Behavior Modification and Implications for Special Education.* Lawrence U of Kansas Pr, 1966.

Harris, A.: *How to Increase Reading Ability* 5th ed. New York, McKay, 1970.

Heckelman, R.: A Neurological impress method and reading instruction. *Acad Ther, 4*(4):277-282, 1969.

Hewett, F.: *The Emotionally Disturbed Child in the Classroom.* Boston, Allyn, 1968.

Hewett, F.: Educational programs for children with behavior disorders. In Quay, H., and Werry, J. (Eds.): *Psychopathological Disorders of Childhood.* New York, Wiley, 1972.

Hewett, F., and Forness, S.: *Education of Exceptional Learners.* Boston, Allyn, 1974.

Hewett, F., Taylor, F., and Artuso, A.: The Santa Monica Project: Demonstration and Evaluation of an Engineered Classroom Design for Emotionally Disturbed Children in the Public School: Phase I: Elementary Level. Final Report. Project No. 62893, Demonstration Grant No. OEG-

4-7-062893-0377, Office of Education, Bureau of Research, U.S. Department of Health, Education and Welfare, 1967.

Hunter, M.: *Teach More-Faster!* El Segundo, Tip Pub., 1969.

Jacobson, E.: *Progressive Relaxation.* Chicago, U of Chicago Pr, 1938.

Jenkins, J., Gorrafa, S., and Griffiths, S.: Another Look at Isolation Effects. *Am J Ment Defic, 76*:591-93, 1972.

Johnson, D., and Myklebust, H.: *Learning Disabilities: Educational Principles and Practices.* New York, Grune, 1967.

Kagan, J.: Reflection-impulsivity and Reading Ability in Primary Grade Children. *Child Devel, 36*:609-628, 1965.

Kagan, J.: Developmental Studies in Reflection and Analysis. In Kidd, A.H., and Rivoire, J.H. (Eds.): *Perceptual Development in Children.* New York, Intl Univ Pr, 1966, 487-522.

Keogh, B.: Hyperactivity and learning disorders: Review and speculation. *Except Child, 38*:101-110, 1971.

Kephart, N.: *The Slow Learner in the Classroom.* Columbus, Merrill, 1960.

Lerner, J.: *Children With Learning Disabilities.* Boston, HM, 1971.

Luria, A.: *The Role of Speech in the Regulation of Normal and Abnormal Behavior.* New York, Liveright, 1961.

Mager, R.: *Preparing Instructional Objectives.* Palo Alto, Fearon, 1962.

Mann, P., and Suiter, P.: *Handbook in Diagnostic Teaching: A Learning Disabilities Approach.* Boston, Allyn, 1974.

Meichenbaum, D., and Goodman, J.: Reflection-impulsivity and Verbal Control of Motor Behavior. *Child Devel, 40*:27-34, 1969.

Myers, P., and Hammill, D.: *Methods for Learning Disorders.* New York, Wiley, 1969.

Nall, A.: What is structured? In Frierson, E., and Barbe, W. (Eds.): *Educating Children with Learning Disabilities: Selected Readings.* New York, Appleton, 1968.

Otto, W., McMenemy, R., and Smith, R.: *Corrective and Remedial Teaching, 2nd ed.* Boston, HM, 1973.

Popham, W., and Baker, E.: *Planning an Instructional Sequence.* Englewood Cliffs, PH, 1970.

Rost, K., and Charles, D.: Academic achievement of brain injured and hyperactive children in isolation. *Except Child, 34*:125-26, 1967.

Schwebel, A.: Effects of impulsivity on performance of verbal tasks in middle and lower class children. *Am J Orthopsychiatry, 36*:13-21, 1966.

Shores, R., and Haubrich, P.: Effect of cubicles in educating emotionally disturbed children. *Except Child, 36*:21-26, 1969.

Siegel, E.: *Teaching One Child: A Strategy for Developing Teaching Excellence.* Freeport, Educational Activities, Inc., 1972.

Smith, R.: *Teacher Diagnosis of Educational Difficulties.* Columbus, Merrill, 1969.

Strauss, A., and Lehtinen, L.: *Psychopathological Education of the Brain-injured Child.* New York, Grune, 1947.

Taylor F., and Soloway, M.: The Madison School Plan: A functional model for merging the regular and special classrooms. In Deno, E. (Ed.): *Instructional Alternatives for Exceptional Children.* Arlington, Counc Exc Child, 1973.

Wallace, G., and Kauffman, J.: *Teaching Children With Learning Problems.* Columbus, Merrill, 1973.

Werry, J.: Developmental hyperactivity. *Public Health Service Grant NB-07347 from NIMH. Pediatr Clin North Am, 15:3,* 1968.

Yando, R., and Kagan, J.: The effect of teacher tempo on the child. *Child Devel, 39:27-34,* 1968.

Volkmor, C., Langstaff, A., and Higgins, M.: *Structuring the Classroom for Success.* Columbus, Merrill, 1974.

SUGGESTED READINGS

Barsch, R.: *Achieving Perceptual-Motor Efficiency.* Seattle, Spec Child, 1967.

Barsch, R.: *Enriching Perception and Cognition.* Seattle, Spec Child, 1968, vol. 2.

Barsch, R.: *A Movigenic Curriculum.* Madison, Wisconsin State Department of Public Instruction, Bureau for the Handicapped, 1965.

Bond, G., and Tinker, M.: *Reading Difficulties: Their Diagnosis and Correction, 2nd Ed.* New York, Appleton, 1967.

Connor, J.: *Classroom Activities for Helping Hyperactive Children.* New York, Center for Applied Research in Education, 1974.

Cruickshank, W., Bentzen, F., Ratzburg, F., and Tannhauser, M.: *A Teaching Method for Brain-Injured and Hyperactive Children.* Syracuse, Syracuse U Pr, 1961.

Della-Piana, G.: *Reading Diagnosis and Prescription.* New York, HR&W, 1968.

Frostig, M., and Horne, D.: *The Frostig Program for the Development of Visual Perception.* Chicago, Follett, 1964.

Gerhardt, L.: *Moving and Knowing: The Young Child Orients Himself in Space.* Englewood Cliffs, P-H, 1972.

Getman, G., Kane, E., Halgren, M., and McKee, G.: *The Physiology of Readiness, an Action Program for the Development of Perception for Children.* Minneapolis, Programs to Accelerate Success, 1964.

Guszak, F.: *Diagnostic Reading Instruction in the Elementary School.* New York, HR & W, 1972.

Hammill, D., and Bartel, N.: *Teaching Children With Learning and Behavioral Problems.* Boston, Allyn, 1975.

Haring, N., and Phillips, E.: *Educating Emotionally Disturbed Children.* New York, McGraw, 1962.

Harris, A.: *How to Increase Reading Ability, 5th Ed.* New York, McKay, 1970.

Hewett, F.: *The Emotionally Disturbed Child in the Classroom.* Boston, Allyn, 1968.

Johnson, D., and Myklebust, H.: *Learning Disabilities: Educational Principles and Practices.* New York, Grune, 1967.

Kephart, N.: *The Slow Learner in the Classroom.* Columbus, Merrill, 1960.

Lerner, J.: *Children With Learning Disabilities.* Boston, HM, 1971.

Mann, P., and Suiter, P.: *Handbook in Diagnostic Teaching: A Learning Disabilities Approach.* Boston, Allyn, 1974.

Myers, P., and Hammill, D.: *Methods for Learning Disorders.* New York, Wiley, 1969.

Otto, W., McMenemy, R., and Smith, R.: *Corrective and Remedial Teaching, 2nd Ed.* Boston, HM, 1973.

Volkmor, C., Langstaff, A., and Higgins, M.: *Structuring the Classroom for Success.* Columbus, Merrill, 1974.

Wallace, G., and Kauffman, J.: *Teaching Children With Learning Problems.* Columbus, Merrill, 1973.

5

Transactional analysis and the management of hyperactivity

Clifton W. Wolf

INTRODUCTION

T HE DEFINITION of hyperactivity in children used in this chapter is as follows: (1) excessive motor activity, (2) disturbance in attention and concentration, (3) poor impulse control, (4) attention-seeking and demanding behavior, and (5) a higher-than-average degree of being refractory to verbal controls and physical punishment. These behaviors, to a considerable degree, interfere in successful academic learning, satisfactory interpersonal relations and an "I'm OK, You're OK" existential position for the hyperactive child.

This paper is not addressed to etiological issues which have been explicated elsewhere, e.g. Birch (1964), Cohen (1967), Schain (1972), Stewart (1970), Tarnopol (1969) and Wender (1971). Treatment for hyperactivity has been primarily drugs and behavioral management as reported in such studies by Barrish (1973), Coleman (1970), Patterson et al. (1965) and Sulzbacher (1972). Simpson et al. (1975), among other studies, question the effective-

160

ness of drugs on the control of hyperactivity. Apparently this issue has not been satisfactorily resolved, particularly in view of better controlled research.

This chapter is concerned with a transactional analysis (TA) point of view of the origins, development and advancement of the script of one who is diagnosed, labeled, perceived or treated as hyperactive with the assumption that the child does indeed manifest the major or agreed-upon characteristics of hyperactivity as reported in the literature.

Berne (1972) and other TA clinicians, e.g. Goulding (1973), Steiner (1971) and Wollams (1973), have studied and reported on two classes of messages given to children—counter injunctions and injunctions. The counter injunctions are generally given verbally and instruct the child on how to make it in life. The injunctions, although given verbally, are frequently given nonverbally through the body language of the parents or other significant adults. These messages are sometimes called *crazy messages* as they interfere, when followed, in healthy growth, development and self-actualization of the young person. These messages may be categorized into being, feeling and thinking injunctions. Examples are "don't be you—be like your sister;" "don't feel sadness—big boys don't cry;" and "don't make decisions—you can't because you have a learning disability."

Admittedly these injunction messages are not always or necessarily given definitively or precisely as the examples above. The relevant attitudes and feelings of these messages from the parents, teachers and others are, however, communicated. The specific shorthand version of "don't be," "don't feel" and "don't think" conceptualize the messages imparted, and they are useful in helping these afflicted ones identify the messages he or she may have used in making lifetime decisions about themselves, i.e. their degree of adequacy, worth and in general their self-image and the manner in which it is to be demonstrated in overt behavior.

In some sense it is a moot question as to whether or not a child is hyperactive. What is important is that he is labeled as such, and this label governs the perceptions, attitudes, feelings and behaviors of others. It is to this issue that TA may help parents and teachers realize that their behaviors, in response to one labeled hyperactive, may do an injustice to the child by giving a message that he or she is not an OK human being with some kind of malady.

The hyperactive child, for example, learns early in life that he is not OK by the manner in which parents, siblings, peers and teachers react to him through negative attention, i.e. negative stroking of his disruptive behavior. A continuation of this reinforcement generally leads to behavior, both inner and outer, indicative of a not OK position. Subsequently, the child makes a decision, either consciously or out of his awareness, that he is not OK, and this decision becomes a self-fulfilling prophecy as the child grows older. Thus, his script advances and he verifies his existential not OK position. The verification of this position involves playing of games, the purpose of which is to have a bad feeling called *racket* in TA terminology. The racket thus is the verification of not being OK.

The use of transactional analysis in the understanding and treatment of hyperactivity in many ways approximates the behavioral management approach as both focus on overt behavior and the environmental conditions that support or extinguish behavior. The behavioral approach is more explicit in specifying the antecedent—subsequent behaviors and TA are more global and historical in conceptualizing the maintenance of behavior. To some degree it also focuses more on intrapsychic behavior when dealing with ego states, games and scripts. A rapproachment between these systems certainly is appropriate.

There is one major drawback to the use of TA with hyperactive children at this time and that is there have been no controlled research studies reported in the literature. All that is available is word-of-mouth reports from clinicians and teachers who have employed it. For this reason, two clinical applications of TA to hyperactivity are reported in this chapter.

AN OVERVIEW OF TRANSACTIONAL ANALYSIS

Eric Berne, who was trained in psychoanalysis, originated transactional analysis based on clinical observations of his patients in individual and group therapy. He created a triparte of the human personality which he referred to as the Parent ego state, the Adult ego state and the Child ego state (see Fig. 5-1). He assumed there are three psychic organs which mediate the organization and implementation of these ego states which he respectively named exteropsyche, neopsyche and archaeopsyche (Berne, 1961).

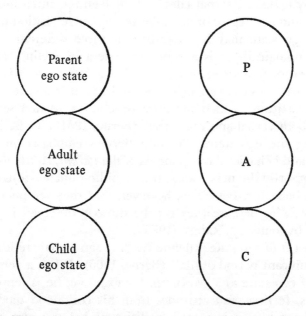

Figure 5-1. The three major divisions of the personality developed by Berne are called ego states and are represented by the above diagrams. The right-hand diagram is an abbreviated representation of the left-hand diagram and is the customary way of indicating the ego states.

Berne (1966) defined an ego state as "a consistent pattern of feeling and experience directly related to a corresponding consistent pattern of behavior." He postulated that the three ego states are not hypothetical constructs as are the terms *id, ego* and *superego* as used in psychoanalysis. These terms represented for him abstractions or inferential concepts whereas his terms *Parent, Adult* and *Child* are experiential and behavioral in nature and involve social realities. Thus, he did not believe his definition of an ego state to be a restatement of Freudian, Jungian or other psychologies. He contended that his definition of an ego state represents conscious aspects of a person's behavior that can be observed objectively in terms of word usage, vocal intonation, body language and how others react to the person under consideration. Additionally, the person himself can detect which ego state is operative by certain internal cues such as feelings, intentions, body language and the degree of muscular tension or relaxation present.

An ego state may be described in three different ways—(1) phenomenologically it is a coherent system of feelings and attitudes relevant to a given situation; (2) operationally it is a set of coherent patterns of overt behavior; and (3) it is a system of feelings and attitudes which motivate or elicit a related set of behaviors, both verbal and nonverbal (Berne, 1961). These levels of describing the ego states illustrate Berne's emphasis on the existential and behavioral components of the *Parent, Adult* and *Child* which comprise the personality, thus avoiding unconscious determinates of behavior. His claim, however, that they are phenomenological realities because they can be directly observed is open to question by some, e.g. Raimy (1975).

The *Child* ego state is defined as ".... an archaic relic from an early significant period of life" (Berne, 1966). When a person is in his *Child* ego state as a grown-up, for example, he is reproducing behaviors, feelings and attitudes from his childhood modified to some degree by his increased facilities of being a grown-up. In other words, his actions and pattern of responses are similar to how he behaved as a youngster. Thus, the *Child* ego state consists of behaviors which are relics of one's own childhood.

The child ego state is composed of two subdivisions, the *Adapted Child* which is externally programmed and the *Natural Child* which is internally programmed (see Fig. 5-2). The former is developed by outside parental-type influences while the latter is free from or attempts to free itself from these influences. The *Adapted Child,* for example, may be compliant, obedient or withdrawn in order to please others as a means of getting along in the world, or it may rebel against forces in the external world. The *Natural Child* acts in whatever ways that please itself and disre-

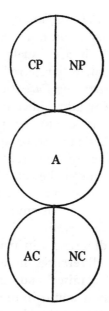

Figure 5-2. Subdivisions of the *Parent (critical parent* and *nuturing parent)* and the *Child (adaptive child and natural child)* ego states.

gards what others think, for example through autonomous acts in expressing creative, angry or affectionate behaviors.

The *Adult* ego state is conceptualized as developing later than the *Child* ego state. This part of the personality is often referred to as a computer as it deals with sensory data and probabilities. Its primary function is to make rational judgments, plan, solve problems and attend to the ongoing requirements of life. Its function is to deal with current realities. In Berne's (1966) definition, the adult is ". . . oriented toward objective, autonomous data processing and probability estimating."

The *Parent* ego state which develops later than the *Adult* consists of a pattern of internal and external behavior learned primarily from one's parents or other significant authority figures. As Berne (1961) stated, it is ". . . a set of feelings, attitudes, and behavior patterns which resemble those of a parental figure." He considered the parent to be divided into two major dimensions—

the *Prejudicial Parent,* or *Critical Parent,* and the *Nurturing Parent* (see Fig. 5-2). The former appears to be composed of arbitrary nonrational attitudes which are usually prohibitive in nature. This ego state is most frequently referred to as the *Critical Parent* in the literature. The *Nurturing Parent* ego state is manifested in love, concern, care and empathy either to self or to others.

Berne also believed that the human personality resulted from the interaction of a few basic drives, or hungers as he preferred to call them, and the influence of significant adults in the life of the developing person. The hungers he considered intrinsic to human nature are those related to stimulation, recognition or stroking; structuring of time; and one's existential position to the self and others. These hungers are organismic in nature and common to humankind. Individual differences in personality functioning are derived primarily from differences in early childhood learning based on how the child was raised, and influenced primarily by his parents and other significant adults in the home, grade school and church. The messages, both verbal and nonverbal, and the kinds of strokes given, both positive and negative, greatly shape the internal and external behavior of the young person.

TA is divided into five major areas of investigation: (1) structural analysis which focuses on the internal and external behavior of the various ego states; (2) transactional analysis which is the analyisis of interpersonal behavior; (3) game analysis which constitutes one type of interpersonal behavior; (4) time structure which involves the different levels of complexity of social behavior concerning stimulation, recognition and stroking ranging from withdrawal to intimacy; and (5) script analysis or the analysis of the overall program one is exhibiting and carrying out from the past to the present to the future. The term *transactional analysis* is used in a generic sense involving all aspects of the system created by Berne and in a specific sense referring to verbal and nonverbal messages sent and received by the various ego states of two or more people involved in interpersonal relations.

Steiner (1974) commented that Berne, aside from his theoretical and therapeutic contributions, made three important assumptions that were revolutionary in psychiatry during the early history of transactional analysis. The first assumption is that people are born OK—that is, they do not come into the world suffering from anything resembling the notion of original sin. It was Berne's contention that, in the form of an aphorism, people are born princes and princesses until their parents turned them into frogs by the way they raised them—that is to say, people do not come into the world with irrational thinking, emotional disturbances or unhappiness. Rather, it is the parents who pass onto their children these conditions. People are at birth and by nature OK. Steiner's (1974) restatement of Berne's position is "Human beings are, by nature, inclined to and capable of living in harmony with themselves, each other, and nature."

The second major concept presented by Berne is that even though people may have mental and emotional disturbances they are, nevertheless, intelligent human beings who are capable of comprehending their issues and the growth process that leads to freedom from that which restricts self-actualization. Furthermore, they must be actively involved in this process even though assisted by one variously referred to as a therapist. In this respect, Berne preferred a conceptual language system couched in nontechnical terminology rather than one obscured by polysyllabic words with minimal common sense referents. His use of the terms *Parent, Adult* and *Child* as the three major components of the personality system is a case in point.

The third major concept is that under the proper conditions of adequate knowledge, motivation and therapist skill, people with functional psychiatric disorders can be cured, not just helped or improved, but cured.

In Steiner's (1974) opinion, these three principles are fundamental to transactional analysis and to those involved in its teaching and therapy. In translating them to an educational setting they are as follows: (1) children are OK even though they behave in ways that deviate from some norm; (2) in spite of the nature of their emotional or behavioral problems they are capable of understanding their difficulties and are to be involved in the resolution of their problems; and (3) they can be cured of their difficulties under proper and adequate conditions.

TA IN THE CLASSROOM

There are a number of TA concepts applicable to the type of classroom atmosphere created and the kinds of behaviors shaped by the teacher and students. Such concepts as ego states, types of transactions among members of the class, games, responsibility, redecision, stroking behavior and basic position illuminate who is doing what to whom, under what conditions and for what reasons.

The fundamental ideas of TA can be taught at least in the upper elementary grades through brief lectures, diagrams and easily-read material (Freed, 1971, 1973). The teacher can give several clear-cut examples of the three ego states and she can have the students practice or try out the inner and outer behaviors of the ego states with each other until cognitive and experiential learning are sufficiently built into the behavior repertoire of the children. Using a tape recorder during a group discussion will illustrate words and voice qualities associated with the ego states. Types of transactions, e.g. *Adult-to-Adult, Parent-to-Child* and *Child-to-Child,* are readily taught through lecture, role-playing, listening to audio tapes and diagrams. In early learning the children can be encouraged to identify the types of transactions, the ego states involved and feelings experienced (see Fig. 5-3).

The concept of responsibility is important in TA. It implies each person is responsible for his own behavior. In teaching this attitude the teacher can set the tone of the learning situation by saying each student is responsible for his own learning and that the teacher is responsible for facilitating this learning. In this frame of reference, if the student needs help he is to ask the teacher for help on a given problem. For example, if a student is having difficulty in solving a math problem, instead of being angry, sulky or timid *(Child* behavior), or critical and complaining *(Parent* behavior), he is to use his *Adult* ego state and request assistance. The teacher, responding from her *Adult,* provides the necessary guidance. If a student does come from *Critical Parent, Rebellious Child* or *Helpless Child,* this can be diagrammed for the student, and he can be asked what is the typical response he generally invites from others and the insuring negative feelings he takes on (racket). If appropriate, the teacher may further explore the issue

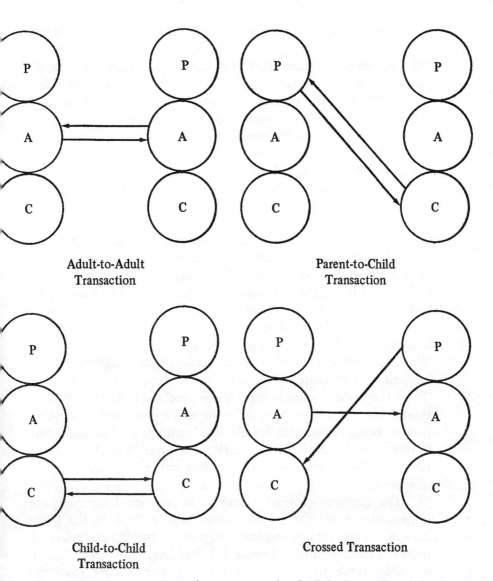

Figure 5-3. Diagrams representing ego states involved in interpersonal behavior between two individuals.

of the ego state used by the student with such questions as "Do you like making yourself upset?" "Do you choose to continue upsetting yourself?" "What other ego state could you use and what do you imagine the results would be?" "Were you to use your *Adult* what might be your options in solving your math problem, e.g. extra help, more study, a simple request for help?"

Assuming the teacher stays in her *Adult* or *Nurturing Parent* rather than her *Critical Parent* or *Adaptive Child* (anxious scared, hurt), as related to the above example, she will not reinforce the negative behavior of the student by giving him recognition through a negative stroke.

A corollary to the concept of responsibility is the idea that people try to rescue others, i.e. do for them what they can do for themselves. In the math example above, if the teacher sees the student squirming, being perplexed, looking around or moving out of his chair in a state of disquietude, she can say in effect, "I see you behaving in such-and-such manner. Are you having a problem? Will you tell me what is your problem? Will you ask me for information as I am here to give you the information you need?" With this approach she directs the student into a different behavior pattern and ceases to respond to his request to be rescued. Thus, the student stops being a Victim seeking a Rescuer and becomes Adult in arranging a different set of consequences appropriate to being responsible for his own learning. Within this frame of reference the teacher stops playing the game "I'm Only Trying to Help You" with consequent frustration, aggravation and weariness.

The patterns of teacher-student interpersonal behavior are subject matter for game analysis. Students, at least in the grade schools, are smaller and less knowledgeable than teachers and come from a Victim position. Teachers, being larger and more knowledgeable, come from a helper position. Our society casts the former in the role of receiver and the latter in the role of giver. Thus, the classroom learning situation becomes fertile ground for the execution of a variety of games, all of which have nothing constructive to contribute to learning and personal authentic satisfaction.

In "I'm Only Trying to Help You" the teacher gives advice, knowledge and homework assignments to the student. If the student plays the companion game of "Look How I'm Trying" or "There's Nothing You Can Do to Help Me," he may defeat the teacher by making excuses or by not following the advice or not completing the homework. At the conclusion of the game the teacher then is entitled to her favorite bad feeling, e.g. frustration or anger. She then can retire to the teacher's lounge and engage in pastiming with colleagues in an "Ain't it Awful" manner, receiving sympathy strokes for her teaching efforts (her Hurt Child is recognized and stroked) or she can pass time in a Critical Parent-to Critical Parent fashion with colleague on how the long-haired generation is going to pot (pun intended). She then can feel justified in her righteous indignation attitude.

According to Berne (1964) the thesis of this game is "Nobody Ever Does What I Tell Them." The aim is to alleviate the teacher of any guilt for the failure of the student to learn properly. The roles in the game involve a helper (teacher) and a client (student). The underlying psychodynamic principle is masochism. The psychological paradigm offered by Berne in terms of ego states is Parent (teacher): "See how adequate a teacher I am," and Child (student): "I can make you feel inadequate." This game enables the teacher to confirm her existential position that people are just ungrateful, which is her motive for the game.

Hyperactive children have ample opportunity for learning the game of "Kick Me," based on the negative attention they receive from unapproved motor activity or acts. The aim of this game is self-castigation and involves a Victim (student) and a Persecutor (teacher, parent, etc.) in which masochism is the psychodynamic principle. Advantages received by the game player are attention through negative strokes from parents and teachers, positive strokes from peers when the behavior displayed is amusing to them and confirmation of a basic position that "I'm not OK."

Other games worthy of the attention of teachers are "Blemish," "See What You Made Me Do," "Why Don't You—Yes But," "Uproar" and "Wooden Leg." Careful attention to the dynamics and maneuvers in these and other games may enable the teacher to recognize how much classroom time is structured with game-playing. Obviously, time spent in playing games is time lost to work activities related to school learning.

The concept of decision or redecision is germaine to people trained in TA. For example, when a teacher has an understanding of game theory and how she uses games as an experiential verification for not being an OK person, she can, if she redecides, stop accepting game invitations from her students by employing the anthesis of the game. Or, when she is aware of setting herself up for a game by offering an invitation to the student to join her in her game, she can become aware of the subsequent forthcoming payoff and decide not to give herself a bad feeling by altering her pattern of behavior. Admittedly, some games are more difficult to recognize in oneself; an involvement in some form of TA group work with a trained TA person will facilitate the necessary self-understanding. Teachers who are versed in game analysis can help each other become aware of the games in their classroom by analyzing the sequence of transactions that occur between them and students. Thus, they will be able to identify the early signs of the game and make appropriate changes in behavior through redecision.

Underlying the behaviors associated with games, transactions and stroking is the concept of basic position. Berne (1961) postulated that people, based on early childhood learning, assumed a basic attitude to self and others colloquially referred to as I'm OK— You're OK; I'm not OK—You're OK; I'm OK—You're not OK; and I'm not OK—You're not OK. These attitudes, or existential positions, influence the developing person, his cognitions, perceptions and feelings and styles of structuring time. The preferred ego states used, the games employed, the trading stamps collected and the types of interpersonal transactions all function in a self-fulfilling manner related to and governed by one's basic position. Thus, the child who plays "Kick Me" from a Helpless Child ego state can invite a teacher to respond from a Critical Parent ego state, collect a resentment feeling stamp which later may be cashed in for a guilt-free outburst in a game of Uproar. In such a series of maneuvers he has gathered enough objective evidence or verfication for a not OK attitude to self and other.

The teacher who accepts the self-fulfilling prophecy of behavior thesis is in a position to recognize the underlying intentions of her students, choose a course of detachment, and not respond in a reinforcing manner to the game invitation.

AN EXAMPLE OF TA APPLIED TO A LEARNING DISABILITY CLASSROOM[2]

The following interview was obtained by the author from a teacher of a learning disabilities classroom. It clearly illustrates the relationship of several principles of TA as applied to classroom teaching and hyperactive children.

Interviewer: Will you give me a brief description of how you use TA as a philosophy in your classroom?

Respondent: The structure in the classroom is the students. I am the facilitator of learning for them, not their teacher. I will be disciplinarian if people choose to break their contract which is "I will not harm others, I will not harm myself. I will operate in such a way that others who choose to learn will not be disturbed."

Interviewer: And this is the contract you have with each student?

Respondent: This is the contract I have with each student. It is an invitation. If they do not choose to do this, they could be transferred to one of the other grade rooms.

Interviewer: You made the contract specifically with each child?

Respondent: Yes. Well, as a group, and then I checked it out with them individually.

Interviewer: Did you have any trouble with this type of contract with your students?

Respondent: I had two students who chose to go into the other classrooms. And their wishes were granted. And there were two students from other classes who came into mine. I have thirty-

---

[2]The interview was obtained from Mrs. Patricia Dickson, Baldwin Park, California.

two students in a portable classroom with no extra facilities, no teacher aids, no extra money.

Interviewer: How has TA helped you in terms of your thoughts about yourself and indirectly your students.

Respondent: I have ceased to be responsible for their learning. If I do not set goals for them, they set goals for themselves. For instance, the first area that I tried specifically allowing students to set goals for themselves was in spelling. At the beginning of each week, the students selected from one to twenty words to learn. There are also some additional words for good spellers which they may elect to choose. When each student has fulfilled the contract, when he has learned the number of words he has chosen to learn and answered the questions in the spelling book, he is through spelling for the week. The students may choose other forms of practice, but I will not give them a test until they have demonstrated that they have completed their task. I have some students who are very slow learners, who have found that answering the questions is too difficult. They prefer memory, so we have worked out a contract, "I will write the words I chose five times before I take the test" or whatever they choose. They take the test, getting all the words perfect, and are finished for the week. Or, they may choose more words after passing the test.

Interviewer: How do you introduce TA to the kids?

Respondent: I use *TA for Kids* (Freed, 1971) in the school library. We talk about warm fuzzies. We talk about having warm fuzzies, needing warm fuzzies, wanting people to have warm fuzzies. So I made some out of fuzzy material one inch square. I told them, "I have only 200 of them. You may choose to do what you wish with them. You may come up and ask for them. The agreement is that the warm fuzzy is a symbol for giving or asking for a stroke." When they come up and say, "I want a warm fuzzy," I say, "Here's a warm fuzzy (handing them one of the 200 made), I love you. It's neat that you came up and asked for a warm fuzzy. It's cool."

Interviewer: What do they do with their warm fuzzies?

Respondent: That was their first question. I said, "It's yours.

You can do with it what you choose." The next question was, "What happens when they are all gone?' I told them,, 'When they are gone I will choose to do nothing about it or will make more. We'll come to that when we get to it."

Interviewer: What did they do when they got them?

Respondent: At the beginning, the students moved around the room, very frequently giving them to others. Some took them home and shared them with their parents. They would come up and slip one into my hand, very secretively, saying, "Here's a warm fuzzy Mrs. Dickson." "Neat! And my warm fuzzy to you is a hug."

Interviewer: That's what the child would say?

Respondent: The child would come up to me, slip the warm fuzzy into my hand and say, "Mrs. Dickson, here is a warm fuzzy." My response was, "That's a neat warm fuzzy. I will give you a warm fuzzy with a hug." Sometimes I would give it back. Or, I would take it and put it in my box. Sometimes I would carry it around and put it in my pocket and they would do the same quite often.

The class progressed. The cloth warm fuzzies were less and less in use, but the stroking continued without the use of cloth warm fuzzies.

Interviewer: Will you tell me more about how you taught your students TA?

Respondent: I spent about ten minutes telling them about having a Parent ego state, how they use their Parent, and giving them one or two illustrations; that they have an Adult that they use to figure things out; and that they have their Child that has fun and feels. Then we practice. It's not a big thing.

Interviewer: What do you mean "practice"?

Respondent: We are going to use them (the different ego states) . For example, in using the Adult ego state I say, "I will share with you when you are in your Adult. Will you share with me any difficulties you are having in your work?" Their nonverbal behaviors sometimes indicate they are frustrated when doing schoolwork. I might say, "Are you using your Adult?" or "Do you need information?" I do not answer questions unless they ask for help, which is another way to demonstrate my own Adult. I will not be a Rescuer and the students know this.

Sometimes the students will say, "I don't understand how to do this" and I'll say, "Oh, You don't understand?" and stop. They soon catch on that if they want help, they ask for it. This way I help them learn to be responsible for their learning. For example, when a new student came into the classroom and she was told that "If you want an answer from Mrs. Dickson, you ask a question."

Initially, when I set up this system of having the students ask for my help, I became anxious and upset because there were so many of them and only me to answer their questions. So I chose not to remain upset (I'm responsible for my behavior just as they are) so I established a market checkout system, i.e. numbers. I have thirty-two students and I have thirty-two numbers (one through 32). If someone wants me, they come up and take the next number off the number rack. When I get to their number, I might say, "I'm yours. What can I do for you?" or "How can I help?" They might say, "Give me a warm fuzzy" or "I want to tell you about my problem. My mother left home last night; I have a new baby brother: I was in such and such; or I had a fight with my brother." Or, "Will you help me find the answer to who was the Revolutionary War general who did. . . .?" I will help them in any way they choose and when they are finished with me I go on to the next student with the next number. I move through my market checkout system about sixty per hour. Sometimes I move slower and it takes two hours to get through thirty-two students. Sometimes a student will anticipate that they need me and will not take the next number up but one, four or five down the line. They are not ready for me at that moment, but they want to be sure when they get ready that I will be there. In this way they learn to plan, anticipate and exercise their Adult ego state in taking care of themselves. They learn very quickly and in this way I am not a Rescuer or a Critical Parent regarding their learning style.

Interviewer: How do you use TA with hyperactive kids?

Respondent: By the students knowing that I respect them and

that they are OK. For example, Charlie,[3] my most hyperactive student, will not sit in his chair for five minutes before moving about. It used to be only two minutes. He would stand on his chair, climb up on his desk, or crawl under his seat. I invited him to do something very physical. Now he goes out and runs around the track in the school yard and comes back in and is able to sit for five minutes and get a lot done in those five minutes. Then it's OK for him to go out and run around again. He learns that he's not an OK person because he's active, and he doesn't have to use his behavior to get negative strokes. He can get warm fuzzies any time he wants them by just asking.

Interviewer: How have you used the TA concept of permission in working with Charlie?

Respondent: At first he was running around in the classroom disturbing the other students. I told him our contract was that he, as with the other students, couldn't disturb the learning of others, and if he wanted to run, he had my permission to run on the track. He doesn't run in the classroom any more or act up in disruptive ways and receive negative strokes from me or the students.

Interviewer: How else do you use permission and convey the idea that the students are OK?

Respondent: Well, for example, I have no rules when and if you can sharpen a pencil. If someone is sharpening a pencil loudly when others are getting instructions of some sort, one of the students will say, "Wait until so-and-so is through. I can't hear." I will wait until that person is through sharpening his pencil. They're OK to sharpen their pencil. I'm no better than they are. That's a neat thing. The result is they will finish sharpening their pencils, they won't be frustrated, and they will have solved the problem. We've waited only five seconds and it takes less time than for me to say, "Will you please sit down and stop sharpening your pencil. You are disturbing the class." It's useful for me.

Interviewer: Do you do any work with the hyperactive kids in terms of what ego state they are in while being hyperactive?

Respondent: Not at first. It's not useful for them until they can control themselves. Usually hyperactive kids have been told

---

[3]"Charlie" is not the student's real name.

it's not OK to be hyperactive. It's not OK to be you. My attitude is they are OK people wherever they are and that it's OK to be themselves.

Interviewer: Does that increase hyperactivity?

Respondent: At first it does.

Interviewer: For how long?

Respondent: Two weeks usually. Then the students themselves learn that they do have power over themselves. It's like, "Wow! If I choose to be quiet five minutes, why don't I choose ten? Is it really necessary to run around the track forty times a day?"

Interviewer: I hear you're doing a lot of decision/redecision work with your permission.

Respondent: I do both. I am helping the students make decisions or redecisions about their behavior. I facilitate their decision-making process. I give them permission to choose and to activate their Adult ego states.

Interviewer: And you talk this way?

Respondent: Yes.

Interviewer: It seems you talk pretty heavy TA language at times.

Respondent: Sometimes.

Interviewer: What else do you do with the hyperactive kid from the TA frame of reference?

Respondent: Give them lots of positive strokes, especially in the classroom setting. They have not gotten positive strokes or they wouldn't have been labeled hyperactive. If parents or teachers think the child is just full of old nick and are really cute in their activity, they are not hyperactive.

Interviewer: That is, they are not labeled hyperactive.

Respondent: Yes. When they are not cute they are labeled hyperactive and they are not given positive strokes.

Interviewer: Berne writes about the four basic positions people assume attitudinally and behaviorally in life, i.e. I'm OK—You're OK; I'm not OK—You're OK; I'm OK—You're not OK, I'm not OK—You're not OK. How has this influenced your behavior as a teacher?

Respondent: Well, for one thing, people sure can shrivel up. I've turned on my Kid (Child ego state.) I was previously a Parent teacher. For example, I would say, "You should . . . . ," "This is where we are. . . .," "This is what I expect next. . . ."—an attitude that "You are the student. You will do what I say. You will follow my rules."

Interviewer: What position were you coming from?

Respondent: I'm OK—You're not OK. And this was not useful. When I was doing behavior modification with them before using TA, I was setting up all the goals and the kids were responding—they were responding because they enjoyed my goals and they liked the reward system, but they were not responding to themselves, i.e. to their own goals. They were not setting their own goals; they were pleasing me.

Interviewer: So you found yourself in an I'm OK—You're not OK position! Then what?

Respondent: Well, I saw them as being OK if—conditionally. And they were OK if . . . I set up neat behavioral goals for them.

Interviewer: Like what?

Respondent: If they followed my goals and stuck to my pattern.

Interviewer: If they did what you wanted them to do.

Respondent: Right. I found out when I started to adopt a TA attitude what I'm OK—You're OK was all about. I had one student who is very much above average and who chose to take one spelling word a week for nine weeks. He finished it on the first day and chose to play. That was my biggest test of me. Is he still OK? And he was still OK.

Interviewer: And what happened to his spelling?

Respondent: After he realized he was OK with me he decided to increase the number of spelling words. He didn't respond previously, however, to the reward system I was using. Nevertheless, I still use behavior mod in the classroom by employing a token system where points are earned for specific classroom achievement that can be cashed in for a reward.

Interviewer: Did the behavior mod program achieve what you wanted from it before you did TA?

Respondent: Yes, it worked before I did TA but. . . .

Interviewer: Why didn't you just stay with it and leave TA alone?

Respondent: Because behavior mod worked only with some students. Those students who, in my opinion, chose not to be OK chose not to get the rewards.

Interviewer: Oh great! Go into that. Stay on that theme.

Respondent: The students who were in the "please me" driver got the rewards and some students chose not to get the rewards.

Interviewer: What ego state were the latter students in?

Respondent: I saw them in their Vengeful Child. They weren't liked by the other students and they "tried hard" to do the work but were unsuccessful. An example is "I studied my spelling words but I didn't learn them—passive/aggressive."

Interviewer: What specific behaviors did you observe?

Respondent: Some would frown, pucker up their lips, look angry or had a whine in their voice.

Interviewer: Let me rephrase this now. In your behavior mod program some kids chose to allow themselves to receive the rewards by conforming to the system. Others didn't. Now, what is the difference between straight behavior mod and the combined approaches of behavior mod and TA?

Respondent: Your formulation is correct. The difference now is that it's OK if they choose not to conform to the reward system. I don't get uptight.

Interviewer: Before you adopted the TA frame of reference I assume you thought that if they didn't buy into the reward system they weren't OK with you. Is that right?

Respondent: Yes.

Interviewer: And did you somehow communicate to them that they weren't OK for not responding appropriately to the reward system?

Respondent: Yes, by giving grades, by calling in a parent for a conference, by sending notes to the school psychologist, by doing all kinds of *neat* things teachers can do to kids. Sometimes by just keeping them in after school.

Interviewer: And now you don't do any of those things?

Respondent: I don't do any of them. What I do is give a certificate at the end of the month that says what such-and-such has done during the month.

Interviewer: I want to check this out. I'm hearing you say that a major dimension that has changed is your going from conditional to unconditional acceptance of the kids. Is that correct?

Respondent: Right on. I'm OK—You're OK.

Interviewer: Regardless of what they do in the classroom?

Respondent: Yes. The neat thing about it is when someone comes up to me and says "This is my assignment, My first question is, "Did you choose it?" They will give me a yes or no. If they choose to do it, I ask them if they will complete it. If they say yes, I ask them what they need from me to help them complete it. What information? One of my phrases is "What data do you need to complete your contract with yourself?"

Interviewer: And they know when you're talking you are coming from your Adult ego state and they from theirs—in other words, an Adult-to-Adult transaction.

Respondent: Right. Again, I tell them I do not choose to be a Rescuer. "When you come to me with a question and you have decided that you need some information I have, you choose to get it. If I were a computer you would come up and push the button and get an answer and you would know what you wanted. I have certain information and you've decided what information you need. You're in charge. How can I help you?" That's the general idea I present. When students come up and say they don't understand, I'll say, "What do you choose to learn?" I'm changing my behavior, not the students' behavior. At least, not in the way I formerly did. They're choosing to learn; I'm not forcing them to learn. I'm the facilitator. And, my discipline problems are minimal since I have worked in the TA frame of reference.

Interviewer: It is evident that you focus a goodly amount of attention on your students being aware of and assuming responsibility for all their behavior. That's one of the cardinal priniciples in TA. Will you elaborate?

Respondent: One girl came to my class from an emotionally

disturbed class in another school district. There was no room in our school for her at the time so I was asked if I would take her. She had rackets (not OK feelings) that were fantastic. Her pick up was, I'm not OK. The only way she could be OK was to play NIGYSOB (Now I got you, you SOB) and she was out to get the teacher. I didn't choose to listen to that. After a short time she escalated to the point where she came up to me, stood in front of me, took a ball point pen, bent it down, broke it in two, and smeared ink all over her face. I looked at her and said, "You smeared some ink all over your face. What do you choose to do about it?" She looked at me and started to cry. Someone else came up to ask me a question and I left her (the one with the ink) at that. She then came back in about five minutes, took a ruler and bit a hunk out of it. She then started to hit someone over the head with it at which point I grabbed her and said, "Your contract to be here is not to hurt anyone. I am aware that you are hurting someone else. Do you want me to take you to the office or do you want to go there by yourself? Do you want me to or will you? You are still in control." I was still holding her forcibly, and she still had the ruler in her hand. She said she wouldn't go down. I remarked that, "Since you won't go down by yourself then I assume you are telling me to take you down. I will take you down." And I took her down.

She came back to class the next day and her behavior was much better. She had not gotten to the point where she was doing any school work although she was able to read. She informed me on three occasions that she couldn't write because she said she didn't know whether she was left or right-handed. I replied, "OK. When you decide what you are, you will write." She said, "I can't write because they don't allow printing in the fifth grade and I can only print. I don't know how to write." I asked her, "What do you want from me? Do you want me to teach you to write? Are you telling me you choose not to write? Or are you saying that you won't write?" "You get me all confused!" "When you're not confused we'll talk again." I went on to someone else.

Interviewer: Beautiful.

Respondent: Two weeks later her grandmother came in and said they had decided to move, that "Something is wrong with my granddaughter." "What's wrong?" I asked. "I don't know. She's not behaving the same. How is she in school?" "She's a nice girl." "You're lying." I said, "I like her." "She's getting along too well. Something is going to happen. She's going to explode. I'm going to take her out of school before she explodes."

I found out the mother was in a mental institution and the grandmother had programmed the granddaughter to go crazy.

Interviewer: Yes.

Respondent: And the fact that she was using her Adult ego state in my class was threatening to the grandmother.

Interviewer: You have given me a great interview. I'm really excited about how you use TA. Thanks a whole bunch.

Respondent: Thank you!

ILLUSTRATION OF TA AND BEHAVIOR THERAPY IN THE MANAGEMENT OF HYPERACTIVE CHILDREN

The following is a portion of a tape recording with a mother who has three children. The ten-year-old son is hyperactive. She was a student in one of the author's TA courses and was readily conversant with TA. The interview begins with the writer and mother discussing the behavioral aspects of her son's hyperactivity.

Mother: Well, if they all are just doing their thing . . . then it becomes chaos.

Interviewer: That is the hyperactivity, and this pouting and getting angry at you and crying and going off to his room is a result of his child or his Hurt Child.

Mother: Yes. I think there is hurt involved there too.

Interviewer: So apparently you have a Critical Parent—Rebellious Child relationship going on.

Mother: "Yes, with him; maybe with all of them and maybe just with the boys. Yeah, I think that is probably true.

Interviewer: And with that knowledge, what can you do?

Mother: Well, move out of my Critical Parent and into my

Firm Parent.[3] Which would, I think, enable me to establish rules and enforce them without feelings.

Interviewer: And what do you mean "without feelings?"

Mother: Without being angry.

Interviewer: O.K.

Mother: But how can I know what kind of rules I can realistically expect he will follow when he is hyper?

Interviewer: What would your Adult say about the kinds of rules you think would be helpful to solving these problems?

Mother: Well, it would seem to me that what bugs me most are the things that I would work on or decide about.

Interviewer: Such as?

Mother: Such as the not sitting still—the wiggling—that's probably number one more than anything. The not eating the food is not the most important thing. With me it is the wiggling. But how do you make somebody not wiggle?

Interviewer: That's a good question.

Mother: My mother sat me on a chair. I was not allowed to move.

Interviewer: Is it important that he not wiggle?

Mother: To him or to me?

Interviewer: To him.

Mother: I'm sure it's not to him.

Interviewer: Why is it important to you that he not wiggle?

Mother: Because it bugs me—it's distracting.

Interviewer: And what ego state are you in when you bug yourself?

Mother: In my Child.

Interviewer: Do you get angry?

Mother: I sure do.

Interviewer: Resentful?

Mother: Umhum.

---

[3]Traditionally, the Parent ego state is divided into two major subcategories, Critical Parent and Nurturing Parent. The author for several years has conceptualized the Parent ego state as consisting of four subcategories, the traditional two plus Firm Parent and Smothering Parent. The Critical Parent is taught as too much Firm Parent and the Smothering Parent as too much Nurturing Parent (see Fig. 5-4).

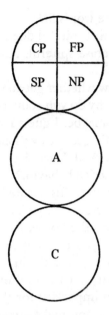

Figure 5-4. Subdivision of the *Parent* ego state into *Critical Parent, Firm Parent, Smothering Parent* and *Nurturing Parent.*

Interviewer: Upset?

Mother: Yes.

Interviewer: And then you come across out of your Critical Parent?

Mother: Yes.

Interviewer: And you let him have it.

Mother: Yes. Then I'm telling him that something he naturally does is not OK and therefore he is not.

Interviewer: That's right.

Mother: Hmmm.

Interviewer: My point of view is that his hyperactivity resides in his Natural Child. He is biologically an overactive person.

Mother: Yes.

Interviewer: You allow your Rebellious Child to get hooked—angry—ticked off—resentful—spiteful.

Mother: Yes.

Interviewer: Do those words fit?

Mother: I don't know if spiteful does.

Interviewer: Then erase spiteful. And then you want to get back at him. Does that fit?

Mother: I don't know whether getting back at him fits.

Interviewer: Then why do you come out as a Critical Parent?

Mother: OK. Yeah—maybe. I guess I see getting back as being an accumulative thing. To get back at somebody—you save it up—you're collecting stamps. And I acted to it. So do I try to limit his behavior? I mean his active behavior?

Interviewer: Do you mean his wiggle behavior?

Mother: Yeah, his wiggle behavior. You know I've moved beyond the table now, into the house. I don't want them to run in the house, they do, but I yell at them for it. I can't stand that. I don't see that as something you do in the house. But maybe I shouldn't limit that activity. At what point do I decide what is important to me that is also important for them to do? Or not do?

Interviewer: I believe you make a compromise. What are the gross behaviors you say to yourself you will not tolerate?

Mother: The running, kicking, throwing the ball. They throw the stuffed animals that can break things.

Interviewer: O.K. What else are gross behaviors?

Mother: Throwing shoes.

Interviewer: Anything else?

Mother: Fighting. I don't care if they yell at one another.

Interviewer: Those are gross behaviors you say you will not tolerate?

Mother: Yes.

Interviewer: And the Adult part says you don't want to tolerate that because of what?

Mother: I don't see these as acceptable behaviors. And they wouldn't do it at school.

Interviewer: That's Parent talking. Go ahead and stay with the Parent.

Mother: Well, there are things that I see that they would not be allowed to do at school. They would not be allowed to do it at other people's homes, in other social situations. They would be allowed to do it outside, but not in a building where there are other people.

Interviewer: Are you making a value judgment that these behaviors will get them in trouble with other people if allowed to continue and that this is not good for them?

Mother: Yes.

Interviewer: And therefore, you want to change these behaviors for their benefit as well as your own?

Mother: Yes. And I can't exist and have any kind of peace and quiet in a home if there are those kind of things going on.

Interviewer: So your Adult says the continuation of these gross behaviors will get these kids into trouble one way or another?

Mother: Yes.

Interviewer: And, therefore, you don't want them to continue.

Mother: Yes, that's true. That has not been the motivation under which I have acted a lot of the time. I have been Critical Parent.

Interviewer: Now, what would your Adult say about the effects of implementing a control program for their gross behaviors? How will the Adult appraise the harmful effects of corralling these behaviors?

Mother: I don't see that there, unless the punishment is worse than the cure, that there could be a harmful effect.

Interviewer: I'm not talking about punishment. I'm just saying the corralling, the stopping.

Mother: I don't see anything wrong with that.

Interviewer: Would it destroy their psyche?

Mother: Not if it's done right.

Interviewer: OK. Do you believe that?

Mother: Yes.

Interviewer: So their giving up these gross behaviors would not be detrimental and damaging. Does your Adult believe that?

Mother: Yes, if it's done correctly.

Interviewer: OK. So now you make a decision. It is OK to bring to an end these forms of gross behaviors.

Mother: Yes.

Interviewer: Do you feel comfortable with that decision?

Mother: Yes.

Interviewer: Will you make that decision?

Mother: OK. Yes—I will.

Interviewer: Say it in a full sentence.

Mother: I agree to limit and put an end to their gross behaviors in the home.

Interviewer: The next question is how to do it.

Mother: Right.

Interviewer: If you come out of your Critical Parent, will that be harmful to them?

Mother: Yes.

Interviewer: In what way?

Mother: Well, because it tells them that they are not OK. That they are not good and valued as people.

Interviewer: When you come out of your Firm Parent, what do you see?

Mother: I can't see Firm Parent as Adult. I don't really experience Firm Parent as being feeling.

Interviewer: The Firm Parent has a sense of power to carry through the decision.

Mother: OK. But it doesn't have a lot of feeling with it.

Interviewer: Only the feeling that you experience when you say "No" in a situation of this kind.

Mother: OK.

Interviewer: Or "I want."

Mother: O.K. I understand.

Interviewer: And were you to come from the Firm Parent, or if you prefer, from the Adult by saying "No" would this be detrimental?

Mother: No.

Interviewer: And going to your Adult, are their options that are available to you in controlling gross behaviors without recourse to the Critical Parent?

Mother: That's very difficult. I tried putting them in their rooms. That worked with some degree of success except that it often means that I have to pick them up and take them there and they are almost as big as I am. I no longer find that effective.

Interviewer: Would you consider using some principle of behavioral management?

Mother: Yes.

Interviewer: Would you consider counting their behavior to get a baseline for a week on a target behavior?[5] The second week, letting them know that you are counting their behavior by posting a piece of paper on the refrigerator and see whether or not the count drops by them being aware of it? And then in the third week, putting a consequence on the behavior when it gets to a certain frequency that you no longer want to tolerate?

Mother: OK. Doing it for each one?

Interviewer: Yes.

Mother: Because I am also thinking about some specific things like making the bed.

Interviewer: That's another issue.

Mother: I mean I will do it. Yes, I will. I count the first week, the second week I post daily how many times they've done it and the third week, at the beginning of the week they get notified of the consequences.

Interviewer: Right. Now, it won't be necessary to use consequences during these first two weeks if the behavior begins to show a drop.

Mother: Do they know the first week I am counting?

Interviewer: No. The first week only establishes the frequency or baseline of their behavior. If they know you are counting that can effect the frequency of their gross behavior. Knowing that you are counting their behavior can have an effect in reducing the frequency of that behavior. At the end of the first week you post the daily frequency count. Then they have a good idea of what they have been doing. During the second week they can see whether or not their behavior is changing. If it drops it is then encouraging for them that they are beginning to take control of their behavior.

----

[5]The mother had previously been introduced to the principle of counting and charting behavior as developed by Ogdon Lindsley.

Mother: OK. What is their motivation?

Interviewer: What is what motivation?

Mother: Their motivation for improving their behavior?

Interviewer: You mean what do they say inside of their head?

Mother: Yes.

Interviewer: I could only guess—I am not certain. It may not even be important if the behaviors drop out.

Mother: O.K.

Interviewer: I assume that they are aware that you don't like it.

Mother: Yes, I would say that they are aware.

Interviewer: I really don't think that question about motivation is important.

Mother: I guess. Except it seems like I don't do things unless I am strongly motivated one way or the other.

Interviewer: There's one way to look at motivation and that's in terms of controlling external events or stimuli that affect another person. For example, there is something about the knowledge of results of one's behavior that influences the changing of that behavior. And the knowledge of results of what your kids do is your posting the frequency of their gross behaviors on a daily basis. The mere fact that they know how often they are doing the thing that they know they shouldn't be doing can be a basis for them making some kind of decision like, "I'm going to stop doing some of this stuff." They have an Adult ego state, and you are providing them data on which to ponder and make decisions. Anyway, just knowing what they are doing can be sufficient for a decrease in their gross behavior.

Mother: OK.

Interviewer: And another thing is the fact that you get out of the game of Uproar or Blemish and you stop giving negative strokes of recognition. They can rip you off for negative strokes for doing things that they know that are irritating to you and thus invite you to structure your time in the game.

Mother: Then like at the dinner table, I count, but we decided that wasn't gross behavior.

Interviewer: But kicking was.

Mother: OK.

Interviewer: Now, since we aren't doing any pure study here of what is effective in bringing about change and what isn't effective in bringing about change, I will give you some general principles. During the first two weeks of counting and thereafter do not yell at them, ever, for their gross behavior. Secondly, give positive strokes for the good things that they are doing. And, if possible, ignore their gross behavior unless it gets grossly gross. In other words, stay out of your Critical Parent and use your Nurturing Parent.

Mother: OK. Then I don't yell.

Interviewer: And what is your reaction to this program?

Mother: Yes, OK. I buy it and I will try it. I will do it. I want to ask you something about James. My second one. He's involved in the first thing (gross behavior), but he has a lot of hostility. James—I see James as a Child—and I really don't know what to do about it.

Interviewer: How does he express his hostility?

Mother: Yells and throws things—he hits.

Interviewer: Those are all gross behaviors.

Mother: Yes.

Interviewer: When he does those things, what do you do?

Mother: James gets much less direct intervention from me than John because he is so spunky. I really tend to do nothing. I ignore him.

Interviewer: Does he show less gross behavior than John?

Mother: It's different. John's is just a random sort of thing. James takes up an enormous amount of psychic space. When he walks into a room, the room has too many people. It is full. Do you know what I am saying? You know, you sense that this kid has power. And I don't object to that. The problem is that I don't know what to do with the hostility.

Interviewer: Well, the hostility that you mention is the gross behavior that you are going to count.

Mother: But there are other times when he gets very angry and just falls apart at something that is not anything specific that I have done, you know, or that because he has been disciplined.

He doesn't like to be touched. Even as an infant. He is extremely hard to love, not in the mental sense of the word, but in the physical sense of the word.

Interviewer: Then give him verbal positive strokes.

Mother: He tends not to take positive strokes.

Interviewer: What does he do with them?

Mother: Ignores them. Or says in a sarcastic manner, "Oh yeah!"

Interviewer: Then what do you do?

Mother: Nothing. In lots of ways, I interact less directly with him than with the other two.

Interviewer: How much positive stroking do you think you are doing with the two boys?

Mother: I try to be conscious of it. I think John gets a fair amount. That's a hard thing for me to judge.

Interviewer: One thing you could do is count your positive strokes. You may need feedback for you as to how many positive strokes you are giving versus how many negative strokes you are giving. This way you will know how often you are Critical Parent vs. Nurturing Parent.

Mother: I find it hard to give strokes only verbally.

Interviewer: Because?

Mother: It just seems like they should be accompanied with a physical gesture.

Interviewer: From an experimental point of view, will you just work on the verbal strokes?

Mother: Yeah.

Interviewer: Particularly since James doesn't like to be touched.

Mother: Why is that? As an infant—that was true from the beginning.

Interviewer: Was he a squirmy kid?

Mother: Yeah—well you know—I breast fed all three of the kids, but James for only two months because he just couldn't stand to be held.

Interviewer: And when you didn't hold him what would he do?

Mother: He was a good baby.

Interviewer: Would he squirm when you weren't holding him?

Mother: No. It was that he liked to get away from it.

Interviewer: Well, holding is a way of confining body movement, which restricts the hyperactive stuff.

Mother: Hmmm. Well, he was much more content with the bottle that he gave himself which bothered me greatly because you know, I just didn't believe in that.

Interviewer: You can give positive verbal strokes without touching, and perhaps this will result in less hostility to your stroking him physically. Because you want to touch is your problem, and in a sense you're laying your trip on him.

Mother: You may be right. I am bothered because he doesn't want me to touch him as much as I want.

Interviewer: What ego state are you in at these times?

Mother: Hurt Child.

Interviewer: You can use your Adult and decide whether it's better to give only verbal strokes, resolve your frustration and have him happier and less hostile, or do what you want by touching and then having him become hostile and you hurt.

Mother: I'm not quite ready to deal with that right now, however I do understand what you are saying. Your point is well made.

Interviewer: And back to the gross behavior issue. . .

Mother: OK.

Interviewer: Will you do the counting and bring it into the group? We'll take it up from there since now you have the basic idea.

Mother: OK. I count the gross behaviors and I count my positive and negative stroking.

CONCLUSION

The values TA has for the hyperactive child or one so labeled and those who work with him are numerous: (1) The parents and teachers have at their disposal a common sense frame of reference and understandable language system that explains their contribution to the maintenance of hyperactivity. It helps them understand the dynamics of the transactions occurring between them and the child and provides them with a graphic presentation (transactional diagrams) as to how they get *hooked* by the hyperactive child. (2) TA teaches how not to get *hooked* by responding from a different ego state. (3) It facilitates a specific and concrete analysis of the games between the adults and the hyperactive child. With these awarenesses the adults can, if they so make the decision, structure their time differently with the hyperactive child, i.e. pastiming, activities or intimacy. (4) Parents and teachers, in studying TA, gain understanding as to how they maintain their own rackets and existential position as they live and work with the hyperactive child. In a TA group situation with parents and/ or teachers focus is directed to their making a redecision concerning their own game-racket-existential position complex. (5) All of the above suggestions apply equally as well to the older hyperactive child when TA treatment is utilized either in individual or group sessions.

In summary, TA provides an understanding of the psychosocial development of a person with hyperactivity or one so labeled, particularly the impact of the verbal and nonverbal messages given by significant adults. The formation of the script and its influence on future behavior as related to hyperactivity are readily explicated. TA offers a treatment frame of reference, both for adults (parents and teachers) and the child, consonant with other established forms of treatment. In this writer's opinion, TA theory and treatment are not at variance with these treatment modalities and can be used adjunctively with them.

REFERENCES

Berne, E.: *Transactional Analysis in Psychotherapy*. New York, Grove, 1961.
Berne, E.: *Games People Play*. New York, Ballantine, 1964.
Berne, E.: *Principles of Group Treatment*. New York, Grove, 1966.
Berne, E.: *What Do You Say After You Say Hello?* New York, Grove, 1972.
Birch, H. G. (Ed.): *Brain Damage in Children: The Biological and Social Aspects*. Baltimore, Williams & Wilkins, 1964.
Cohn, R.: The neurological study of children with learning disabilities. In Frierson, E. C., and Barbe, W. B. (Eds.): *Educating Children with Learn-*

ing Disabilities: Selected Readings. New York, Appleton, 1967.

Coleman, R.: A conditioning technique applicable to elementary school classrooms. *J Appl Beh Anal, 3:*293-297, 1970.

Freed, A. M.: *TA for Kids.* Sacramento, Jalmar, 1971.

Freed, A. M.: *TA for Tots.* Sacramento, Jalmar, 1973.

Goulding, R.: New directions in Transactional Analysis. In Sager and Kaplan (Eds.): *Progress in Group and Family Therapy.* New York, Brunner-Mazel, 1973.

Patterson, G. R., Jones, R., Whittier, Jr., and Wright, M. A.: A behavior modification technique for the hyperactive child. *Beh Res Ther, 2:*217-226, 1965.

Raimy, V.: *Misunderstandings of the Self: Cognitive Psychotherapy and the Misconception Hypothesis.* San Francisco, Jossey-Bass, 1975.

Schain, R. J.: *Neurology of Childhood Learning Disorders.* Baltimore, Williams & Wilkins, 1972.

Simpson, R., Reece, C. A., Kauffman, R. E., and Jones, F. C.: The effects of Central Nervous System Stimulants in Classroom Behavior of Hyperactive Children. Unpublished manuscript, Kansas City, University of Kansas Medical Center, 1975.

Steiner, C. M.: *Games Alcoholics Play: The Analysis of Life Scripts.* New York, Grove, 1971.

Stewart, M. A.: Hyperactive children. *Sci Am, 222:*94-98, 1970.

Sulzbacher, S. I.: Behavior analysis of drug effects in the classroom. In Semb, G. (Ed.): *Behavior Analysis and Education,* 1972.

Tarnopol, L.: *Learning Disabilities: Introduction to Educational and Medical Management.* Springfield, Thomas, 1969.

Wender, P. H.: *Minimal Brain Dysfunction in Children.* New York, Wiley-Interscience, 1971.

Wollams, S. J.: Formation of the script. *Trans Anal J, 3*(1):31-37, 1973.

6

Reflection-impulsivity and information-processing from three to nine years of age[1]

John C. Wright and Alice G. Vlietstra

COGNITIVE STYLES or conceptual tempos have received considerable attention in developmental psychology journals in the past decade. In particular, reflection vs. impulsivity, though by no means a new idea, has served as a rallying point for those who are fleeing from the abuses associated with IQ tests but who are committed to the notion that children learn and think differently, and that working with them as unique individuals in all kinds of settings where learning is supposed to take place is a superior strategy to that of treating them all alike. The problem, of course, is that the flight from one system of stereotypy for tagging individuals may well lead to the creation of a new one, with all the dangers attendant thereto.

It appears that labeling a child as hyperactive, minimally

[1]This research was funded by the National Institute of Education under a contract with the Kansas Center for Research in Early Childhood Education No. NE-C-00-3-0104. Opinions expressed are those of the authors and do not necessarily represent the opinions of the sponsoring agency.

brain damaged, autistic or impulsive is in principle just as likely to lead to rigid tracking in school, self-fulfilling prophecies, diagnosis by syndrome rather than open-ended experimentation and the like, as is labeling him dull-normal, deprived or culturally disadvantaged. The purpose of this paper is to suggest a possible exception to this gloomy pattern of escaping one rigid taxonomy only to perhaps unwittingly give birth to another.

One thesis of this paper is that reflection-impulsivity, together with information-processing efficiency (sometimes called ability or even intelligence) serve jointly to describe the speed and accuracy of information-processing more comprehensively than either style or ability alone, and more effectively than the raw speed and accuracy data on which their diagnosis is based.

A second thesis of this chapter is that while reflectivity may be both preferred by the dominant culture and correspondingly more useful than impulsivity for survival in that culture, it is nevertheless likely that certain important but educationally neglected forms of intellectual competence develop more fully within the impulsive mode. Moreover, both in terms of the maintenance of cultural pluralism and for the sake of broadening the range of individual intellectual competence it appears desirable to help each child function well in both modes and be able to determine which is the more effective in any specific information-processing situation.

Thirdly, we hope to show that of all the information-processing domains involved in thinking, it is the selection of stimulus inputs and the organization of information acquisition that is primarily related to individual differences in cognitive style.

Approximately 150 publications and presentations have appeared as of the fall of 1974 on conceptual tempo (reflection vs. impulsivity), and the pace is accelerating. There are two likely reasons for the popularity of the topic. One is a general increase in concern for taking account of the individual variability among children in how they learn and take in information, with an eye to the effective individualization of instruction within homogeneous groups differing in cognitive style. The other appears to be the emerging centrality of reflective vs. impulsive patterns of processing information as regards attention, exploration and search behavior.

OVERVIEW

We begin with the assumption that basic cognitive development is a real but not directly observable process that takes place in basically the same form but at different rates and with different styles and emphases in different individuals. While the development of underlying intellectual competence is not directly measurable, the emergence of specific sequences of abilities, always dependent in part upon the tasks used to assess them, always influenced by the relevant environmental history of learning experiences, and always colored by individual styles and abilities is nonetheless observable. Most of the literature on individual differences in thinking has been concerned, of course, with assessment of developmental status (mental age) and with the rate at which development has progressed (IQ).

One of the many domains in which intellectual development has been charted is of special relevance to a consideration of the origins and importance of cognitive style. That domain is the development of information-getting behaviors in general and, in particular, the developmental trend from stimulus-controlled exploration to logic-controlled search. In another article (Wright and Vlietstra, 1975) the writers have argued that there is such a developmental trend, that it is based in part on the child's growing familiarity with more and more of his environment, and that the evolution of passive exploration into organized search is a critical component of the development of basic information-processing competence. Since the acquisition of orderly information from the environment is a necessary precursor to effective thinking, reasoning and problem solving, it seems reasonable to look to the domain of attention for signs of the earliest differentiation of individual styles of thinking.

Specifically, we have been struck by the frequency with which identifiable age changes in how children explore, scan or search their stimulus environment is paralleled by identifiable individual differences in children's stylistic preferences or modes for processing information. We suggested (Wright and Vlietstra, 1975) that the more primitive mode of attention, which we call exploration, is distinguished by a number of salient properties. First of all, it occurs in younger children. It is seen mostly in relatively unfamiliar situations. It is disconnected, transient, playful in nature. It appears to be controlled more by physically salient and attention-getting features of the environment than by purpose or logic. It thus lacks continuity or selectivity based on informativeness and is guided by a process of serial habituation of attention to the most novel, salient or inherently interesting features of the environment at any moment. It is basically comprised of rapid, automatic responses to only the most obvious stimuli present.

By contrast, search behavior as we have defined it is a later development ontogenetically and also occurs later than exploration in the microhistory of a child's encounters with any particular situation or task. It thus occurs in more familiar settings and is better internally organized and more coherent, persistent and goal-directed. Search resembles work more than play and is controlled primarily by the intentions of the child, by clear expectations of the consequences of actions, and by the logical constraints of the situation or task as they are defined by the child himself. Thus, search is active where exploration is passive. The child engaged in search is therefore better able to overcome the effects of differences in stimulus salience and to selectively attend to stimuli more in terms of their relevance to his ongoing instrumental activity. Finally, it is characterized by deliberate slowness, sequential continuity and logical convergence.

While these descriptions emerge from the literature on attention and information-getting in children, it is interesting to note how closely they resemble differential descriptions of the information-processing characteristic of children who differ in cognitive style, and it is to that parallel that much of this chapter is addressed. In particular it appears that exploration is often characteristic of the information-getting of impulsive children while search behavior resembles that typical of reflective children.

Following a review of cognitive style in conceptual and

methodological terms, the chapter reviews the influence of cognitive style on individual differences in information-getting behavior in general, and attention in particular. The style variable of interest is reflection vs. impulsivity, which consists of a set of preferences, abilities and biases that are in principle orthogonal to general intellectual ability or cognitive efficiency, but which emerge as consistent approaches to information-getting and processing within individuals in the early childhood years and which generalize across many tasks and situations. As conceptually defined, impulsives are relatively fast but error prone, while reflectives are slow but accurate in task where speed and accuracy are negatively related.

This crystallization of a characteristic style in each child appears to occur earlier in girls than in boys. It appears to interact with other aspects of cognitive development (indexed by age) in the acquisition of systematic search behavior—that is, impulsives at any age seem more responsive to perceptually salient features of the environment than are reflectives, who in turn appear more advanced in the development of systematic search.

Correspondingly, reflectives are credited with superior visual analysis skills and often appear superior on performance measures of intelligence, though impulsives are sometimes judged more expressive, fluent or creative. Thus, the apparent developmental superiority of reflectives over impulsives is repeatedly confirmed in both logical information-getting and cognitive performance, but it appears that it might be fairer to characterize impulsives as being more curious and exploratory than as in some normative sense attentionally and cognitively slower to develop. Analogously, the very reflective child might be viewed as resisting socialization pressures to risk error in the service of speed, and as clinging to a redundant, exhaustive and even compulsive set of safe search routines beyond that point of declining uncertainty at which they become no longer functional.

HISTORY AND METHODS

The general notion of cognitive styles has been a periodic concern in the cognitive literature and in studies of the effects of personality on perception and thought. Typically, styles have been described either as offshoots of differential abilities tests (Witkin, 1964) or as cognitive correlates of basic personality characteristics (Frenkel-Brunswik, 1949). Often, a typology or syndrome has been named, given an operational definition and correlated with other personality and cognitive measures. Such distinctions as broad vs. narrow categorizers (Bruner, Goodnow and Austin, 1956), automatization (Broverman, 1960), intolerance of ambiguity (Frenkel-Brunswik, 1949) and ego-controls (Gardner, Jackson and Messick, 1960) have been studied primarily in adults.

Two major bodies of research in this area have focused on the development of individual styles and abilities in children— the work of Witkin and that of Kagan. Witkin (1964) has devoted many years to the study of field dependence-independence, field articulation and the general problem of psychological differentiation. While the operational definitions employed have been primarily performance on perceptual tasks, the developmental theory has been thoroughly grounded in a general theory of psychological development which, like that of Heinz Werner (1961), goes far beyond the perceptual-cognitive patterns used to define style.

Like the Witkin group, Kagan and his associates have developed first a perceptually-based dimension of cognitive style (Kagan, Moss, and Sigel, 1973), then extended it in a revision to incorporate more cognitive aspects (Kagan, Rossman, Day, Albert, and Phillips, 1964). Their first approach was to assess cognitive style by the nature of the process and criteria used to categorize stimuli taken from the Make A Picture Story (MAPS) test. This led to the development of the Conceptual Style Test (CST) for assessment of analytic vs. nonanalytic attitudes in school-age children and adults (Kagan, Moss, and Sigel, 1973). The task involved grouping any two of three pictures together and giving a verbal rationale in support of the grouping. Responses were scored as analytic-descriptive (the category of interest) or one of two forms of global (nonanalytic) response—categorical-inferential and functional-relational. Rather soon after developing the CST, Kagan and his colleagues began to note that analytic responders not only attended to specific, concrete details in the pictures, but took more time to complete their groupings. Indeed, it seemed that they were often almost compulsive in their painstaking attention to detail, while global responders tended to provide rapid if sometimes superficial responses based more on immediately salient features of stimuli than on an analysis of perceptible details. The correspondence of this distinction to that made by White (1965) between the temporal zones of automation and decision should be apparent.

Accordingly, the second generation of Kagan's work has been focussed on a variable dubbed *conceptual tempo,* or a distinction between reflective and impulsive responding which is based on both the speed and accuracy with which a child can complete match-to-sample problems on a test called the Matching Familiar Figures test (MFF). It is noteworthy, first, that this test clearly has a correct answer and an implication that both speed and accuracy are important to good performance unlike previous procedures which were more open-ended and preferential; second, that the MFF is scored on the basis of the child's choice in a trade-off decision between speed and accuracy rather than as a power test of speed plus accuracy. That is, the MFF assesses not only whether a child is relatively fast and accurate vs. slow and inaccurate (in this sense it could be used as a power test), but given a necessary choice, whether the child emphasizes speed at the expense of accuracy or the reverse.

When Kagan (1964, 1973) first proposed conceptual tempo as an important dimension of cognitive style, he was clearly within the tradition of Witkin, Gardner, Frenkel-Brunswik, Broverman, Luchins and many others who sought to chart the no-man's-land between testable personality traits and testable intellectual abilities. Unlike most of them, however, he employed a two-dimensional rather than a scalar frame of reference. He argued that on any task containing sufficient response uncertainty, important individual differences between fast, inaccurate and slow, accurate responders could be detected, differences which generalized broadly enough across tasks and endured long enough in individuals to warrant terming them conceptual style or tempo and identifying the children as impulsive and reflective, respectively. Examples of MFF items are shown in Figures 6-1 and 6-2. The test has been used mostly with school age children, and the task is to identify as quickly and accurately as possible that figure

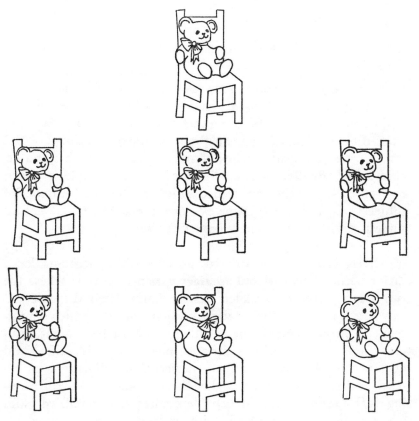

Figure 6-1. Sample MFF Item.

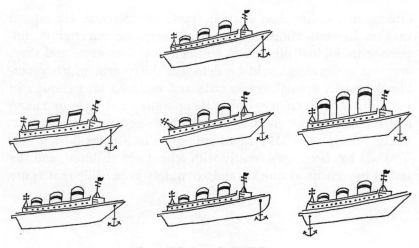

Figure 6-2. Sample MFF Item.

in the array of six which exactly matches the standard at the top.

Empirically Kagan used a scatterplot of time to first response against number of errors, using median cuts on each population studied to establish the four quadrants of the scatterplot—fast and error-prone (impulsive), slow accurate (reflective), fast and accurate, and, finally, slow and inaccurate. An example is shown in Figure 6-3. He then proceeded to ignore the small number of subjects who fell in the latter two quadrants. Many, but not all subsequent investigators have done likewise.

There appears to be an axis of reflection-impulsivity along which children can be ordered, an axis which accounts for a major portion of speed and accuracy variance on tasks where the two are negatively correlated, less variance when they are uncorrelated, and very little variance when they are positively correlated. This conclusion suggests that a task analysis might be in order and that the off-axis variance needs to be identified and documented. Moreover, at least on verbal intelligence tests, reflectives do not score much higher than impulsives, yet the growing R/I literature consistently deprecates the impulsive child while often concerning itself with ways to make him more reflective.

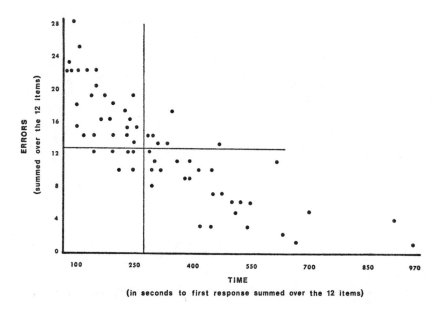

Figure 6-3. Sample scatterplot of MFF time against errors (After Nelson, 1968).

EXTENSION TO PRESCHOOLERS: THE KRISP

Since Kagan's MFF does not appear to work as well with children younger than six to eight years, i.e. error scores are very high, rate of response is constrained, and the negative correlation between speed and accuracy declines, we have developed a parallel instrument for children from three to eight years old called the Kansas Reflection-Impulsivity Scale for Preschoolers (Wright, 1971b) or simply the KRISP. The Kansas Center for Research in Early Childhood Education has administered the test to more than 900 preschoolers throughout the United States and in six foreign countries. A *User's Manual* (Wright, 1973) has been published, and a series of technical reports are available from the author.

The KRISP is also a match-to-sample test but with somewhat simpler items (Figs. 6-4 and 6-5 are examples). It has two equivalent forms, showing fairly good agreement in time and error

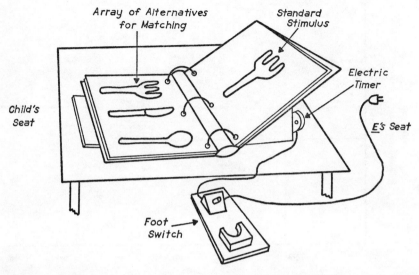

Figure 6-4. Apparatus for administration of the KRISP, showing practice item.

scores and very good agreement in assignment of children to the four quadrants of the speed/accuracy scatterplot. User norms are presented graphically so that the dual criteria of speed and accuracy can be used simultaneously. Figure 6-6 is an example. Retest reliability is also highly satisfactory, but there is a practice effect which shows up as sharply reduced errors and slightly *increased* time to respond on the second administration, regardless of which form was used first. With five and six-year-olds the KRISP agrees well with the MFF in assigning children to quadrants.

Over longer intervals (c. one year) girls show high stability of relative scores from age three on. Boys, however, do not appear to stabilize until four or five years of age. By stability, of course, we mean relative standing within a short-term longitudinal sample since each group shows an age-related trend toward sharply decreasing errors and slightly increasing times. We shall return to a consideration of the significance of the developmental trend later.

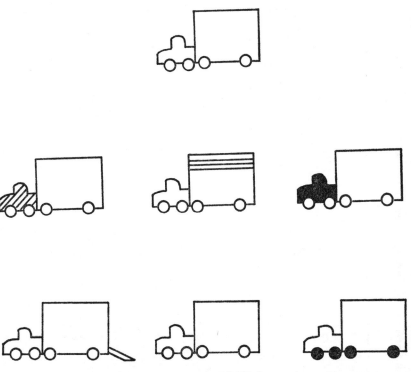

Figure 6-5. Sample KRISP Item.

The relationship of KRISP scores to other tasks is fairly consistent but with exceptions which again depend upon the presence of and relationship between speed and accuracy within the task in question. For example, impulsives have a higher general activity level and a slightly shorter mean attention span during individual work time in the preschool. Reflectives are slower and more complete in their drawings on the Bender Gestalt test. In a draw-a-line-slowly task the reflectives are able to inhibit movement better when so instructed but also make more jerks and stops despite instructions to minimize them. On a motor coordination task (the Fisher-Price Tumble Tower®) reflectives take slightly less time to completion than impulsives, but the task is so structured that every motor error requires additional

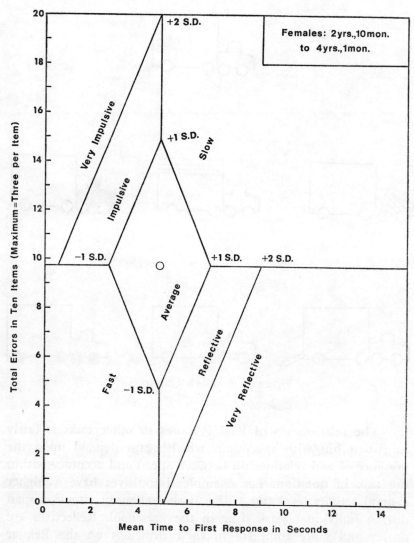

Figure 6-6. Sample page of KRISP norms from *User's Manual*.

time to correct so that speed and accuracy are positively correlated in that task.

Finally, in problem-solving tasks, reflectives show more evidence than impulsives of developing a systematic strategy, con-

fining their attention to relevant cues, and overcoming the effects of stimulus saliency when it inheres in irrelevant cues.

NATURE OF COGNITIVE STYLE: ABILITIES AND PREFERENCES

Although theoretical discussions of cognitive style have long pointed out their special status as lying somewhere between intellectual abilities and personality characteristics, containing some elements of both, Kagan's conception of tempo permits one to derive a more precise formulation of the relationship between style and ability. By his (1964) definition, both speed and accuracy on a test such as the MFF are inherent in the conceptual model. That is, reflectives are defined as those subjects scoring both above the median in time to first response, and below the median in total errors. Conversely, impulsives are defined as both faster and more error prone than the median scorer in their peer group. When speed and accuracy are negatively correlated on any task, median cuts of the time vs. errors scatterplot yield most reflectives and impulsives, and relatively few fast-accurate and slow-inaccurate responders. The tasks which produce such scatterplots of time against errors are those with a high degree of response uncertainty, which according to Kagan is necessary if the task is to differentiate reflectives from impulsives. In more general terms, it is hypothesized here that there is a class of tasks having a relatively large number of initially promising solutions or having an attractive or dominant initial response which is likely to be incorrect. Such tasks tend to be those on which speed and accuracy are negatively correlated, and which therefore contain more variance between impulsive and reflective responding than between efficient (fast-accurate) and inefficient (slow-inaccurate) responding. Any such task should be appropriate for distinguishing conceptual tempo and correspondingly inappropriate for assessing ability or efficiency.

Conversely, there exists a domain of tasks on which the primary difficulties consist not in stimulus or response selection as on the MFF, but in the planning, monitoring and execution of a sequence of steps with orderliness and precision. In this second class of tasks the defining attribute is that speed and accuracy are *positively* correlated. This may be because fast, automatic, associative responders are usually correct, because each error requires the retracing of previous steps, thus consuming more time, or because slow responding produces an increased strain on memory which leads to more errors. A scatterplot of time against errors on such a task would produce a large number of efficient (below the median on both variables) and inefficient (above on both) responders, but the off-quadrants containing reflective and impulsive responders would be more sparsely populated by definition. Such a task would be an appropriate *power test* for efficiency but would not elicit sharp differences between reflective and impulsive responders.

In principle, the decision as to whether to emphasize speed or accuracy is orthogonal to the *abilities* of the child. It is on many tasks a stylistic and strategic rather than a capacity-based decision. But having argued that preferences are fundamentally involved, one must at once acknowledge that on most learning tasks differential utilities are attached to speed vs. accuracy as criteria of performance. On a vast majority of learning and problem-solving tasks the fast-accurate performance is clearly preferable to the slow-inaccurate one. But, conversely, on almost any task, especially when speed and accuracy tend to be negatively correlated, the major difference variance is between fast-inaccurate responders (impulsives) and slow-accurate responders (reflectives).

Most studies of the correlates of reflection-impulsivity have found reflectives in one way or another to perform better than impulsives. In general, this trend may be taken either as evidence against the assumption that conceptual tempo is orthogonal to efficiency or ability, or for the proposition that our culture values accuracy over speed in most situations where a trade-off is possible. That reflectives typically behave in ways that resemble chronologically older children while the performance of impulsives often resembles that of younger children has been established for a number of different kinds of tasks. In defense of the cultural value interpretation, however, it may be argued that the majority culture trains and maintains through differential reinforcements that which it values. In a culture that values reflectivity the precocious social learned will thus acquire reflective behaviors sooner and also demonstrate his precocity in other domains while the child who is socialized more slowly will perhaps display more impulsive behaviors and frequently appear less mature in other domains as well.

There are a number of indicators of superiority on the part of reflectives over impulsives when other indices of intellectual development are used. For example, Wright (1973) indicates that older impulsives resemble younger reflectives on time and error scores. Both educable and trainable retardates appear impulsive in relation to their age/sex peers. Most such relationships appear to be more a function of accuracy than of speed—that is, increased errors in younger children and retardates are not always accompanied by reduced time scores. Nevertheless, reflectivity is only slightly positively correlated with verbal IQ. Moreover, while certain performance measures of intelligence such as the WISC picture arrangement appear to strongly favor reflectives over impulsives at all ages studied, verbal IQ such as that obtained from the PPVT shows a much stronger differentiation of the off-quadrants (fast-accurate scoring higher than slow-inaccurate) than between reflectives and impulsives.

Perhaps because of the value placed by Western culture on accuracy and convergent, *correct* response, most of the correlates of conceptual tempo seem to show the cognitive superiority or greater intellectual maturity of reflectives as compared with impulsives. Impulsives are more hyperactive and have poorer motor control (Bucky, Banta, and Gross, 1972; Campbell, 1973; Campbell, et al., 1971; Harrison and Nadelman, 1972; Loo and Wenar, 1971; Meichenbaum and Goodman, 1969; and Sykes, Douglas, Weiss, and Minde, 1971). Intellectually and educationally disadvantaged children appear more impulsive than their respective control groups (Duckworth, 1972; Errickson and Wyne, 1972; Hallahan, 1970; Lewis, Rausch, Goldberg, and Dodd, 1968; Schwebel, 1966; Singer and Smith, 1974; Stevens, Boydstun, Ackerman, and Dykman, 1968; and Zucker and Stricker, 1968).

Correspondingly, impulsives tend not to perform as well as reflectives in both intellectual ability and educational achievement (Cathcart and Liedke, 1969; Coop and Sigel, 1971; Kagan, 1965b, 1965c; Keogh and Donlon, 1972; Messer and Damarim, 1970; and White, 1971).

Impulsives are more socially responsive (Farley and Farley, 1970; Ruble and Nakamura, 1972; and Strommen, 1973) and are either more or less anxious than reflectives, depending upon whether one assesses generalized anxiety or fear of failure, respectively (Campbell and Douglas, 1972; Chiu, 1972; Kagan, 1965a; 1966c; Messer, 1970; Reali and Hall, 1970; and Sigel, 1965). Impulsives are poorer on certain standard laboratory tasks such as Piagetian conservation (Fleck, 1972), decentration (Shine, 1971), discrimination learning (Hemry, 1973; Massari and Schack, 1972; and Odom, McIntyre, and Neale, 1971), reasoning (Kagan, Pearson, and Welch, 1966a; Kagan, et al., 1964; McKinney, 1972, 1973; and Yando and Kagan, 1970) and memory (Messer and Damarim, 1964 and Siegel, Kirasic, and Kilburg, 1973).

In free play situations reflectives carry on more different activities simultaneously, have longer attention spans, spend less time in transition, and are less mobile and less dependent on the teacher than are impulsives (Welch, 1973). Second grade teachers rate impulsive boys as less task-oriented and considerate than impulsive girls, while impulsive girls are rated as more distractible than reflective girls (McKinney, 1974).

It is argued here that reflection-impulsivity is or should be so measured as to be as nearly orthogonal to ability or intelligence as possible. This would mean that in power tests where speed and accuracy are positively correlated and the major variance is between the fast-accurate and slow-inaccurate quadrants, reflectives and impulsives should have approximately the same distribution of scores. On style or preference tasks, however, this assumption (or definition) would mean that the major variance between reflectives and impulsives would result from a choice or strategy rather than from differential ability or efficiency. In such a task as the MFF the child is instructed to be as fast *and* accurate as possible. The structure of the task permits, nay forces him to choose between the more or less mutually exclusive strategies of maximizing speed at the expense of accuracy or taking as long as may be necessary to be error-free. Therefore, some of the general superiority attributed to reflectives in the literature may result from the strong bias in our culture, and particularly in our educational community, toward emphasizing accuracy over speed whenever the two are in conflict. It is easy to defend this bias in our system on a number of rational grounds, but our purpose is neither to attack or defend it, but to explore some of its implications for children.

Reflectives undoubtedly have a hard time making decisions when the criteria are unclear. One would expect them to develop a lower tolerance for ambiguity than impulsives and to be generally less expressive and fluent in situations where uncritical productivity of ideas is required. Reflectives should be poorer at brain-storming, estimating and guessing, and inventing new solutions to problems than are impulsives. We have as yet no persuasive data to support this conjecture, but neither do we have any evidence to the contrary. Among school age children fluency and expressiveness are probably more characteristic of impulsives than of reflectives as seen perhaps in divergent thinking or the various creativity measures that have been developed for children. In school settings impulsives should show no disadvantage and perhaps superiority in dance, drama, art, story-telling and creative writing. On the other hand it would be surprising if reflectives were not superior in most aspects of the traditional core curriculum.

While the culture of middle America has probably pressured the impulsive child toward being more careful and cautious, and, to a lesser degree, the reflective child toward greater alacrity and decisiveness in responding, there is some evidence that the urban poverty cultures selectively reinforce quick and clever responding more than deliberate and considered thinking. Moreover, there is at least one piece of evidence (Briggs and Weinberg, 1973) that by school age, children have already conformed to societal pressures not to respond too quickly or too slowly and have developed some resistance to yielding further to the norm of expected behavior. The evidence takes the form of a finding that it is easier by training to speed up impulsives and to slow down reflectives than it is to slow down impulsives or speed up reflectives, despite the fact that statistical regression worked directly against that outcome.

All of these considerations should make us cautious about assuming either that impulsives are less likely to learn without difficulties in school than reflectives, or, by the same token, that special training and remediation are more needed for impulsives than for reflectives. It can be just as debilitating to learning and intellectual development to be obsessively concerned with detail and unable to make up one's mind as it is to jump to conclusions and guess carelessly. Does this mean that educators should be striving to make everyone fast and accurate at all times and to constrain that variance which is a matter of style and preference rather than efficiency or ability? This conclusion, too, has a serious drawback. To attempt systematically to constrain the stylistic variance in any population of children by moderating the impulsivity of impulsives and the reflectivity of reflectives is to suppress the individual quality of a child's thinking in order allegedly to optimize his efficiency and performance. We need somehow to protect the spontaneity of impulsive thought and impart some of it to the reflective child for use in appropriate circumstances. Correspondingly, we need to value the ruminative quality of reflective thought and help impulsive children to achieve it in situations where it is effective.

EFFICIENCY AND TEMPO: A NEW MODEL AND DIAGNOSTIC PROCEDURE

In response to the lack of any standard way of using the MFF and the initial success in standardizing the KRISP, and in response to the problems involved in merely tagging or categorizing children as *reflective* or *impulsive*, Salkind and Wright (in preparation) have developed a new scoring procedure. Some of the problems raised in an article by Block, Block and Harrington (1974), which was critical of the MFF, may also be resolved by taking a fresh conceptual definition for which the new scoring procedures are appropriate.

This model (Wright, 1974) makes one basic assumption—that reflection-impulsivity and cognitive efficiency are inherently uncorrelated with one another. Figure 6-7 is a hypothetical scatterplot of mean time to first response against total errors on any task, regardless of the task-determined correlation between latency and errors. Both axes have been standardized in terms of z scores. A pair of orthogonal axes has been drawn rotated forty-five degrees from the empirical axes about their common mean. These rotated axes represent style dimension (impulsive to reflective) and an efficiency dimension (fast-accurate to slow-inaccurate), and are in principle independent of one another as indicated by their orthogonality. Individuals are identified by transforming their time and error scores to z scores and plotting their location on the scatterplot. Their style and efficiency scores are then derived graphically by dropping perpendiculars from their data point to the rotated axes, appropriately scaled.[2] Data points and their reflections (dotted lines) on the rotated axes are shown for seven hypothetical individuals.

In practice virtually all tasks would have some variance associated with each of these rotated axes—that is, there would ordinarily be some variance attributable to conceptual efficiency (upper-right to lower-left axis in Fig. 6-7) and some attributable to cognitive style (upper-left to lower-right axis). It is proposed here that such a schematic conceptualization will serve to clarify the discussion of conceptual tempo, which must otherwise be awkwardly discussed in terms of stereotypic prototypes (*the reflective* or *the impulsive*), or at the empirical level must be described by two scores, time and errors, neither of which alone directly taps the variable of interest.

Note (in Fig. 6-7) that the stippled area is plotted to indicate

---

[2] Impulsively is defined as $I = Z_{errors} - Z_{latency}$. This I-scale has a mean of zero, and positive scores are impulsive; negative scores are reflected. Efficiency is defined as $E = Z_{errors} + Z_{latency}$. This E-score also has a mean of zero, but positive scores indicate inefficiency (slow-inaccurate) while negative scores are efficient (fast-accurate).

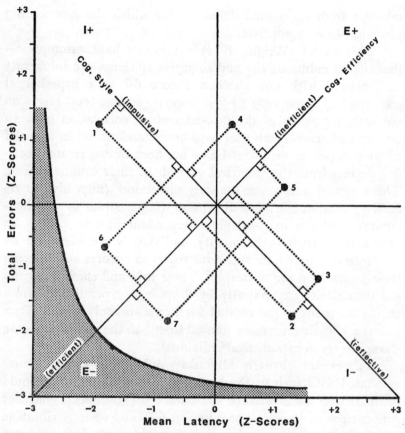

Figure 6-7. Hypothetical time and error scores showing rotation of axis and derivation of *I* and *E* scores.

that for any task there are some limits to efficiency—that is, it is in principle impossible always to respond with zero latency and perfect accuracy. The shape of the curve indicates, however, that a strategic trade-off is always possible. One can respond almost immediately if accuracy is of no concern, and, conversely, if one is willing to take long enough, he can be virtually assured of a correct response. On most tasks, however, there are some constraints of both kinds, and the strategic decision of the subject really amounts to weighing subjectively the utility of being speedy versus that of being confidently error-free. It is this decision, however implicitly made, that distinguishes typically reflective from typically impulsive responders.

Persons 1 and 2 (see Fig. 6-7) clearly differ in cognitive style with 1 being impulsive and 2 reflective, but they differ hardly at all in efficiency; they are both more efficient than the average of the norming population. Persons 2 and 3 are both about equally reflective, but 3 is not as efficient as 2. Persons 4 and 5 are both inefficient, perhaps of below-average ability, but even in the slow-inaccurate quadrant where they both fall there may be important stylistic differences to be taken into account. Of the two, 4 is somewhat more impulsive and 5 is somewhat more reflective. Analogously consider persons 6 and 7. By this model they are about as impulsive and reflective as were 4 and 5 respectively, but they are both about as efficient as the task permits.

Finally, it should be noted that gains in efficiency as a result of training need not attenuate individual differences on the style axis. To construct differential training procedures for individual children, one might consider a plan for reflective subjects 2, 3 and 5, following the Premack principle that made access to un-hurried tasks on which they presumably do better and which they probably prefer, contingent upon meeting a sliding speed cri-terion on a rapid, fluent production task. Conversely, an appro-priate procedure for impulsive subjects 1 and 4 would be to make access to a speed-based guessing game contingent on their meet-ing an accuracy criterion on convergent tasks that is set just beyond their current performance level. Hopefully such proce-dures would increase both the flexibility of stylistic strategies employed and teach children to discriminate among settings and tasks in which impulsive and reflective styles are most appropri-ate. After all, the long-range goal is still to give each child the widest possible range of information-processing skills and to teach him when to use each of them, while simultaneously preserving the uniqueness and individuality of his intellect.

PERCEPTUAL EXPLORATION AND SEARCH BEHAVIOR

While reflectives are possibly more mature and successful than impulsives in a variety of convergent tasks and problems, a somewhat clearer picture of that superiority results from comparison of the different modes they use in generating and selecting information from the environment. The preponderance of evidence to be reviewed below suggests that the major difference between impulsives and reflectives in information-processing is rooted in the patterns of exploration and search that predominate. Impulsives engage in perceptual exploration and scanning that are more focussed on salient cues, are more distractible, especially by irrelevant social stimuli, and are more reward than information-oriented. Reflectives, in contrast, appear better able to decenter attention, to select relevant and informative stimuli, to process information in logically ordered sequences, and to engage in generally more systematic search. To the extent that reflectivity, like efficiency, generally increases with age, this aspect might be referred to as an ability. But any potential advantages of being impulsive, such as creativity, fluency and expressiveness, may be buried beneath the culturally preferred attributes of precision and accuracy. Moreover, regardless of age trends, reflectives and impulsives appear to maintain their relatively distinctive conceptual styles over time. It may therefore be wise to continue to regard reflection-impulsivity in part as a stylistic preference as well as a differential ability variable.

The study of the developmental trend from exploratory, playful observing behavior toward deliberate and systematic search (Wright and Vlietstra, 1975) has identified a number of properties of scanning behavior on which reflective and impulsive children differ. It is hypothesized that impulsive responding characterizes information-getting performance where the salience of environmental cues and automated responses predominates. Impulsive responding in this sense is associated with exploratory attending patterns. Conversely, reflective styles of response not only characterize older children and involve more systematic and logical patterns of search behavior, but also, like effective search, they require more task than stimulus orientation and more fully-developed schemes for performing cognitive operations. In capsule form, it is suggested that impulsive responding, like passive exploration, is perceptually organized and predominates in less familiar tasks and situations whereas reflective responding, like systematic search, is cognitively organized on the basis of established operative concepts.

Drake (1970), using Mackworth's (1967) method, recorded the visual fixations of impulsive and reflective third graders and college students while they performed a modified MFF test. During the first six seconds of performance on the MFF items, reflective children and impulsive adults allocated to the standard a significantly larger portion of their fixations and looking times than did the other two groups, i.e. impulsive children and reflective adults. Younger impulsives failed to appreciate the logical centrality of the standard while adult reflectives systematically scanned the array to isolate variable features which could then be checked easily in the homologous part of the standard. In terms of response time the reflective subjects looked at a larger portion of all stimulus figures and in more detail than did the impulsive subjects. Reflectives also made about twice as many homologous comparisons (successive fixations of corresponding parts of different figures) as did impulsives. Consonant with previous research on reflection-impulsivity, adults appeared more reflective than did the children. In particular, it is noteworthy that adults compared a larger number of design features across figures and repeated these comparisons more than children. In other words, they were more systematic and exhaustive in their scanning.

Siegelman (1969) investigated reflective and impulsive observing behavior in fourth grade boys using a button-pushing response. The MFF test was presented in an apparatus constructed so that the child had to push a button in order to make each figure come into focus. Reflective children looked more frequently and spent more time looking at both the standard and alternative stimuli than did impulsive children. Impulsive children spent proportionately more time looking at the standard stimulus, the eventually chosen alternative, and the longest observed stimulus than did the reflectives. In other words, impulsives were more biased. They tended to favor a few alternatives and choose between them, whereas the reflectives observed more of the alternatives and distributed their attention among them in a more homogeneous and systematic fashion.

Siegelman hypothesized that there was a broad difference in the search strategy for the two types of subjects. She suggested that the reflectives differentiated the properties of the array by comparing the alternative for explicit differences and consulting the standard for confirmation, selection and elimination. This was an efficient algorithm for this task. Siegelman further noted that impulsives appeared more likely to compare the standard globally with one alternative at a time, interpreting the task as a series of up to six binary decisions (*same* or *different*). As soon as they failed to find a difference between an alternative and a globally memorized standard, they chose that alternative (1969). Again, the impulsive child appeared to behave like the younger child in terms of his inability to develop a systematic strategy for effective search.

In summary, the age change from partial, passive and erroneous scanning in young children to more exhaustive, active and systematic search in older children is paralleled in the differences between the scanning strategies of impulsive and reflective children at a single age level.

Ault, Crawford and Jeffrey (1972) included the off-axis quadrants—that is, children who were fast-accurate and those who were slow-inaccurate—in a study of visual scanning during administration of the MFF. Reflective and fast-accurate nine-year-olds made more systematic and exhaustive comparisons than did impulsives and slow-inaccurate responders. Wright (1971a) used the Kansas Reflection-Impulsivity Scale for Preschoolers (KRISP, Wright, 1971b) to identify reflective and impulsive three and four-year-olds. Unlike Siegelman's (1969) nine-year-olds, among the preschoolers it was the reflectives who paid most attention to the standard stimulus. Apparently heavy attention to the standard is a strategy developmentally intermediate between nonsystematic scanning (young impulsives) and differentiation of alternatives (old reflectives). Both young reflectives and old impulsives appear to operate at this intermediate level.

McCluskey and Wright (1975) compared the visual fixation and scanning behaviors of reflective and impulsive preschoolers as selected by the KRISP. The children were given a task in which they had to find the locus of a single difference between two otherwise identical pictures. The stimuli were designed so that a record of portions fixated could be made and so that the difference never appeared in certain places. Fixations of these regions of the two figures were designated *uninformative comparisons.* Reflectives made more homologous comparisons, defined as successive fixations on the corresponding parts of the two figures, than did impulsives. Furthermore, a higher percentage of the reflectives' homologous comparisons were directed to informative regions than was the case with impulsives. Additional main effects favoring older preschoolers over younger ones and females over males were obtained. There were no significant interactions involving age, sex or style. Once again, maturity of information-getting behavior is implicated as the explanation for the superiority of reflectives over impulsives.

Kagan (1966b) has found that children who are impulsive on the MFF respond to salient stimulus dimensions whereas those subjects who are reflective tend to be visually analytic and to search for relevant cues whether they are salient or not. The attentional strategy of the impulsive child resembles that of the centered young child. He may take one quick glance at a stimulus and thereby be more likely to pick up color cues than form cues which require more extensive scanning. On this basis, Katz (1971) hypothesized that reflective children would show more form preferences than impulsive children. Color-form preferences were investigated in impulsive and reflective children ranging between three and five years of age. Three stimulus series which varied with respect to the relative salience of color and form cues were used. The results showed that reflective children made more form responses to all stimuli than did the impulsive children. Moreover, reflectives had longer response latencies and made more comparison glances between the stimuli than did impulsive children.

CONCEPTUAL STRATEGIES

Just as reflectives and impulsives differ in visual scanning as an index of information intake at the perceptual level, so also do they differ in the strategies they employ in logical search or problem- solving tasks. For example, McKinney and Banerjee (1974) found that the impulsive fourth graders solved fewer concept formation problems than reflectives when no memory aids were provided, but the difference disappeared when the children were allowed to keep track of those instances on which they had received feedback by removing them from the array.

Consistent with previous findings concerning cognitive style differences, Siegel, Kirasic and Kilburg (1973) found that reflective preschoolers performed better than impulsives on a recognition task, regardless of whether the items were designed to benefit from verbal labeling, visual feature analysis or both. This finding again implicates attentional and perhaps other nonverbal differences in processing favoring reflectives, whose visual search has been shown to be more systematic and exhaustive.

By a training and transfer procedure, Odom, McIntyre and Neale (1971) were able to assess the actual information being processed and learned by reflective and impulsive kindergarteners. They found that only the reflectives responded in a way that indicated they were processing feature differences in the stimulus arrays. From their data, it appears to us that the impulsives assumed that any transfer item having the same standard sitmulus as a remembered training item must be identical to that previous item, and thus made more errors than the reflectives, who proceded with less confidence and more caution and skepticism.

Massari and Schack (1972) used a two-button task in which the *correct* button and the *incorrect* button were positively reinforced on 70 and 30 percent of the trials, respectively, (condition CP) or in which the correct and incorrect responses were negatively reinforced, i.e. punished, condition CN, on 30 and 70 percent of the trials, respectively. In addition, they sampled their first grade male subjects on the basis of cognitive style, half the subjects in each condition being reflective, and half impulsive. As predicted, impulsive boys were more reinforcement-oriented and tended to maximize positive reinforcement in condition CP more than did the reflective subjects who displayed more complex patterns. Condition CN introduced costs and risks that led the reflective children especially to slow down their rate of response and utilize still more complex response sequences, apparently in an attempt to minimize losses. Again, it appears that reflective children, like older children generally, tend to organize information-processing more carefully and extensively than do impulsives, especially when a need for caution is indicated in the situation. Under such conditions we suggest reflectives do not simply test more complex hypotheses derived by intuition and hunches. That would be an appropriate strategy for older impulsives or for anyone under low-risk conditions. Rather, it is suggested that the complex patterns observed in reflectives under condition CN suggest an enhanced concern with orderly and systematic search across the logically possible alternatives, much as the observing responses of reflectives were relatively systematic and exhaustive in the Siegelman (1969) and the Ault et al. (1972) studies cited above.

Adams (1972) confirmed these results with six-year-olds, but not with eight-year-olds in a replication of Weir's (1964) three-button probability learning task (two buttons were never reinforced; the third was reinforced on a 33 percent random reward schedule —VR-3). The six-year-old reflectives responded like Weir's seven and nine-year-olds, using left-middle-right search strategies while the young impulsives followed the win-stay, lose-shift strategy characteristic of five-year-olds in Weir's study.

In a simple concept formation task McKinney (1972) found that twice as many school-age impulsives as reflectives used a mixed or random strategy of selecting instances from a matrix to test for concept membership while more than twice as many reflectives as impulsives used the maximally efficient and sophisticated focussing strategy. Analogously, Nuessle (1972) employed a concept identification procedure to demonstrate that reflectives, like older children in general, were proficient focussers and took relatively long times to process feedback before the next response as compared with impulsives and younger children. Delay following feedback was in general positively correlated with proficient focussing.

Both Ault (1973) and Denney (1973) have demonstrated the superiority of reflectives over impulsives in a twenty-questions game where the more efficient strategy is to ask constraint-seeking (categorical) questions like "Is it a tool?" rather than hypothesis-seeking (guessing) questions like "Is it the rake?" The Denney study further demonstrated that tempo is involved in the selection of a querying strategy by showing experimentally that instructions to hasten responses increased the number of hypothesis-seeking questions.

TRAINABILITY OF COGNITIVE STYLES

It is useful to examine the cognitive-style training studies to determine the extent to which the variables that control exploration and search also control performance differences in conceptual tempo. One variable that has been hypothesized to control exploration and search is the presence of logical cognitive strategies and constraints. If so, providing impulsive children with verbalized logical strategies may result in more reflective behavior. Correspondingly, the removal of logical, cognitive constraints should produce more impulsive and exploratory responding. Since responses in the cognitive mode take more time, forcing a reflective individual to respond faster should result in more exploratory and impulsive behavior. These hypotheses may be examined by investigating the results of studies that have attempted to modify conceptual tempo. The cognitive training studies have either manipulated the speed of the response by reinforcement (Briggs and Weinberg, 1973), provided training designed to induce systematic scanning or more cognitive control over performance (Egeland, 1974; Heider, 1971; Meichenbaum, 1971; and Meichenbaum and Goodman, 1971), or used a model to demonstrate an impulsive or reflective conceptual tempo (Debus, 1970; Denny, 1972a; Kagan, Pearson, and Welch, 1966b; and Ridberg, Parke, and Hetherington, 1971).

Briggs and Weinberg (1973) trained groups of reflective, impulsive and neutral fourth grade boys to speed up or slow down their response by giving them reinforcement and prompts based only on their response latencies to previous items. The training procedures were effective in changing latencies (both upward and downward) as well as the error scores for all three groups of subjects in training as well as on an immediate posttest even though reinforcement had been contingent only on latency. Training generalized to the subjects' later performance on a WISC picture arrangement subtest, but not to their performance on additional perceptual motor tasks. In a second experiment on the effects of various types of task incentives and reinforcement Briggs and Weinberg did not find reinforcement so effective. Reinforcement changed latencies during training but not on an immediate MFF posttest.

A number of studies have attempted to change an impulsive conceptual tempo by introducing more cognitive control either by direct training of a strategy for systematic scanning or by training impulsives to verbally instruct themselves. One difference between impulsive and reflective children on the MFF test is that impulsives do not examine the array of alternatives as carefully as reflectives. Nelson (1968) taught fourth grade boys a method for making visual comparisons typical of naturally reflective subjects of that age. The training procedure was effective in producing the appropriate changes in speed and accuracy on an immediate posttest (Nelson, 1968), but not when the subjects were retested six months later (Wright, 1972).

Heider (1971) compared the effect of increased reinforcement incentives for accuracy, enforced delay of response and instructions containing an explanation of an appropriate task strategy among impulsive seven-year-old, middle and lower-class boys. For the lower-class children only, task strategy instructions significantly reduced errors and increased latency of response.

The reinforcement procedure, again only for lower-class children, increased response latency but had no effect on errors. Egeland (1974) compared the effectiveness of systematic scanning training and delay-of-response training on changing an impulsive conceptual tempo in second graders. Both groups showed significant increases in response time and decreases in errors relative to a control group on an MFF test given immediately after training. In addition, subjects given training in systematic scanning maintained the changes in response time and errors on a delayed posttest two months later. The group given delay-of-response training maintained the change in response time but showed an increase in errors. Training also generalized to tests of reading, especially for subjects given training in systematic scanning.

Meichenbaum (1971) and Meichenbaum and Goodman (1969) found that impulsive children verbalize significantly less than reflective children and have less verbal control over their behavior. In an ensuing study Meichenbaum and Goodman (1971) trained impulsive second grade children to talk to themselves in an attempt to increase self-control. Impulsive subjects trained to verbally instruct themselves became significantly more reflective in their responses than did control subjects on an immediate MFF posttest as well as on several other measures of generalization. In another study Michenbaum (1971) compared the effects of modeling combined with self-instruction and modeling alone. Modeling alone was sufficient to slow down the impulsive child's response time for initial selection, but only with the addition of self-instructional training was there a significant decrease in errors. These changes in latency and errors were maintained on a follow-up test one month later.

Other studies have attempted to induce more efficient scanning strategies by changing the stimulus materials. Zelniker et al. (1972) gave impulsive and reflective children a match-to-sample task where five of the alternatives were identical to the standard and only one differed. This task is different from the usual MFF, where the alternatives differ and only one is identical to the sample. After ten differentiation items, impulsive subjects made significantly fewer errors on an immediate MFF test. The procedure had no effect on latency of response.

Ridberg et al. (1971) investigated the effects of a model on the modification of conceptual style. They exposed impulsive and reflective fourth grade boys to a filmed model displaying a response style opposite to their own cognitive style. Following exposure to a reflective model, impulsive children showed a significant increase in response time and also made significantly fewer errors. The changes were stable over a period of one week. The cognitive style of the reflective children was only partially modified by exposure to an impulsive model. While there was an increase in errors, which was maintained for a week, reflective subjects tended to show an unexpected increase in response time. Other research using modeling techniques has not been as effective. Debus (1970) had third graders observe reflective models or models with contrasting or changing patterns of response. He found a significant effect of a reflective model in changing response latency but not errors. Moreover, the effects were not stable. Only girls who observed change models maintained significantly greater latencies than control subjects on a delayed posttest two and one-half weeks later. Kagan, Pearson and Welch (1966b) also used a modeling procedure with impulsive subjects and obtained an effect on latency but not on errors.

In summary, the training procedures that have produced the most enduring changes in latency and errors have been those which were designed to elicit more cognitive control over behavior either through self-instruction procedures or training in systematic methods of processing the information in the task. This effect would be predicted from an exploration-search framework whenever longer times and fewer errors are the desired outcome since they are manifestations of logical search as well as criteria of reflection. Procedures involving stimulus manipulations such as those of the Zelniker et al. (1972) study and the modeling studies were not as effective as those of the training studies in that they produced changes primarily in latency. These results can be interpreted in the exploration-search framework as producing delayed response in impulsives by manipulation of stimulus salience, to which they are particularly sensitive, without effective change in information-getting strategy where their deficit is greatest. Because salience-based treatments did not elicit primarily cognitive control, they did not produce as strong effects as the strategy-training procedures. Finally, reinforcement has been shown to be more effective in changing a reflective conceptual tempo than in changing an impulsive one. At the least this is consistent with the contention of the exploration-search hypothesis that task-related information such as reinforcement has a greater impact than stimulus salience for reflectives while the reverse is true of impulsives.

In an ingenious training and transfer study, Zelniker and Oppenheimer (1973) trained impulsive kindergarteners either to concentrate on matching similarities or to concentrate on differentiating distinctive features of stimuli. In transfer either the standard stimuli were the same but the variants new, or the variants were the same and the standard stimuli new, or as a control both were new. Matching emphasis in training facilitated a strategy of memorizing the prototype (standard) while differentiation emphasis in training facilitated the better strategy (in terms of error reduction in transfer) of distinctive feature analysis. Clearly the latter is preferable when one is seeking to help impulsive children be more analytic.

With regard to more abstract logical strategies such as those involved in the twenty-questions game discussed above, Denney, Denney and Ziobrowski (1973) attempted to increase the frequency of constraint-seeking behavior, a strategy characteristic of reflective and older children, by various modeling techniques with six-year-olds. Where a previous study had obtained no modeling effects at this age (Denney, 1972), this study did obtain such effects. Either modeling of an elimination strategy or modeling of a successively larger array were effective, the former more so with girls and the latter with boys. Although the subjects were not selected on the basis of reflection-impulsivity, their age insured that their approach to the problem resembled that of somewhat older impulsive children, and the success of the treatment method might well generalize to such a population.

Since retarded children have in general showed a tendency to score as impulsive on either the MFF or the KRISP, it is of practical interest to know whether training techniques designed to encourage various aspects of reflective responding are helpful when applied to retarded children. Lowry and Ross (1974) used a period of enforced delay of response in a receptive-language, color-discrimination task and demonstrated large improvements with delay as compared with no-delay controls. The study used only a small number of the most impulsive children in a sample of severely retarded children, and to that extent generalization of the powerful findings must remain limited pending a replication.

Denney (1973b) has published an excellent review of the literature on the training of information-processing styles, tempos and strategies up to that time, and there is appended to this chapter a nearly complete bibliography of cognitive style and conceptual tempo studies up to November, 1974.

SUMMARY AND CONCLUSIONS

We began with the hope that assessment of individual differences in cognitive style, especially reflection-impulsivity, might provide descriptive but nonevaluative data about how children process information. We suggested that the most germinal place to look for such differences was in the information intake behaviors characteristic of young children in relatively unfamiliar settings. In particular a parallel was drawn between the impulsive-reflective continuum and the evolution of attending from exploration to systematic search. We countered the clear implication that impulsive children are developmentally inferior to reflective ones by suggesting that the difference is in part a product of cultural bias and in part a consequence of the kinds of tasks used to assess cognitive style. A review of some of the literature on reflection-impulsivity showed repeated examples of cognitive superiority of reflectives in terms of performances valued by the culture on tasks it defines as relevant, even when the analysis was extended to younger children than are usually studied in the cognitive-style literature.

An alternative conceptual model and scoring procedure was described which is designed to assess reflection-impulsivity as a continuous dimension on which each test administration yields a numerical score in place of a categorical tag, and one which is designed to ensure that cognitive style is assessed in such a way as to be maximally independent of cognitive efficiency or general intellectual ability.

Finally, a review of the literature on attentional patterns and conceptual strategies of reflective and impulsive children demonstrated that different parameters describe their information-getting behavior and that different kinds of antecedents control that behavior and may be used to modify it. Exploratory behavior, quite likely motivated for the most part by curiosity, evolves both maturationally and as a consequence of the increasing familiarity of a variety of task settings into systematic and strategic search. Correspondingly, there are developmental changes in the performance of children on cognitive-style tests such as the MFF or the KRISP from less mature performances which would be diagnosed as indicating impulsivity had they occurred in an older child to more mature performances which would be classified as reflective in a younger child. But despite the overall normative change with increasing age from impulsive-like behaviors toward reflective ones, the relative standing of individual children on the R-I dimension appears to be fairly stable over time.

We may conclude that individual differences in cognitive style in part reflect, as does tested intelligence, differences in the rate of progress through a developmental sequence common to most children. To the extent that intelligence is identified primarily as cognitive efficiency whereas style more nearly reflects strategic habits and preferences our conception of impulsivity as orthogonal to efficiency may be useful both in designing individualized curricula tailored to the child's particular style, and in prescribing the kinds of information processing skills whose acquisition would most broaden each child's general intellectual competence.

APPLICATIONS

The systematic application of what we have learned about information-getting and information-processing in reflective and impulsive children of various ages must await a period of evaluation research and the development of differential treatment techniques. The classroom teacher as well as the school psychologist can probably identify the most reflective and impulsive children intuitively, and it may not be particularly helpful to have MFF or KRISP test scores except as a confirmation of intuitive judgment.

The availability of numerical scores for impulsivity and efficiency, independent of one another as proposed above, may prove to be an improvement on the gross tagging of children as *reflective* or *impulsive*. Ideally a classroom teacher could place each child on a scatterplot such as that in Figure 7, normed on a larger comparable sample, and could thereby obtain a more comprehensive graphic summary of where each child was in relation to all the others. Such a class plot could, for example, help a teacher decide whether the deficiencies characterizing a particular child's typical performances are more a matter of inefficiency or of impulsivity. If inefficiency is the culprit, we have no indication of a particularly preferred remediation strategy other than reinforced practice, but if what might have passed for low ability or inefficiency is in a particular child more appropriately diagnosed as impulsivity, then we make some tentative guesses as to the kind of help that would be most effective.

To the extent that more serious educational problems appear to be encountered among impulsives than among reflectives, such as their hyperactivity and short attention span, certain general strategies of remediation are apparent from the information summarized. One is to start early the process of identification and remediation of extreme impulsivity. Preschool is not too early an age to begin to identify impulsivity and to differentiate it from inefficiency or low ability. Another is to maintain consistent but noncoercive training over a relatively long period of time in small doses since heavy, short-term intervention seems to have results with limited generalization and durability. Both styles do work for the child to some extent, producing at least a certain amount of success and satisfaction and a corresponding resistance to change. Thirdly, it has been repeatedly demonstrated in the research literature that impulsives lack an ability not only to perform detailed analysis, but more specifically to discriminate what is task-relevant from what is merely salient, interesting or novel. Therefore, continuous emphasis on a goal orientation, attention to relevant cues and continuity of effort (such as planning methods to keep track of what has been done and what remains to be done) are all indicated as potential contributors to the effectiveness of a training program.

More specifically, three strategies stand out as most promising. One is to concentrate training and practice (with the usual ingredients of modeling and reinforcement) on teaching the child to differentiate the perceptual environment more carefully, focussing on small and nonsalient cues that are nevertheless critical in a discrimination or matching task. Games in which things that are superficially identical prove on closer inspection to have nonsalient but critical differences would be examples of such practice tasks.

The second strategy might be to set up work sessions in which deliberate slowness is suggested, modeled and differentially reinforced. Praise, points, tokens or access to a new task might be made contingent on a child's taking longer to respond on the training task, provided, of course, that the additional time is spent in concentrated attention to the materials.

A third strategy for working with impulsive children would be to concentrate on information intake decisions, attention, selection of information sources or loci, and development of question-asking skills including those involved in talking to oneself. In such exercises, success and approval would depend upon the child's asking informative, relevant or convergent questions;

looking selectively at relevant cues; or consulting less salient but more appropriate sources of cues in the task environment.

Each of these strategies might be incorporated within an individualized remedial program as well as being used separately or in combination for selected groups in the classroom. One possibility for an individualized program would be to determine which activities an impulsive child does well and enjoys, and to reinforce and encourage the abilities involved such as self-expression in humor, music, drama, dance, story-telling, art and the like. Impulsives usually have some special abilities and preferred activities which up to a point should be made a source of pride and satisfaction to them. Having identified and strengthened such domains of rewarding activity, the teacher might then gradually require higher and higher standards of both quality and quantity in performance on one or more of the training exercises suggested above as ways of earning access to those activities which the impulsive child does best and enjoys most.

Analogously, the reflective child, though clearly less handicapped in this culture by his preferred style than is the impulsive, can under certain circumstances be limited in the kinds of intellectual activities he can enjoy and excel at. Just as the hyperactive and disruptive, acting-out child is more likely than the withdrawn and anxious child to be seen as a problem by the teacher and to receive some kind of individualized assistance, so the very reflective child is less obviously limited by his style in intellectual growth than is the impulsive child, and may as a result be relatively neglected.

Remedial activities for the very reflective child would ideally be designed to encourage not only freer and more fluent behavior in the expressive domains where the impulsive child presumably functions best, but also in such problem-solving skills as estimating, intuiting, guessing, imagining and other task-related skills where preliminary or approximate responses are required, and where the task involves conditions of high uncertainty, more than one solution, inadequate time or information, little redundancy or confirmation, and/or a probabilistic outcome. Correspondingly the reflective's skill and patience at convergent analysis and attention to detail should be prized, but also practice and success at imaginative, expressive and intuitively-based information-processing tasks and games should be made the necessary behaviors upon which permission to indulge and exercise the reflective bent is made contingent, at least during periods devoted to individually prescribed work.

We may speculate that impulsives are more playful, curious, socially responsive, exploratory and attentive to salient stimulus features of the materials they work with, and therefore the sensorily rich and most manipulatable features of remedial task materials should be emphasized for them. Reflectives, however, are generally more responsive to the logical requirements of a task, its goals and purposes, and the demonstrably different levels of effectiveness in achieving them offered by different coherent strategies verbally presented.

We end as we began, with a warning. The aim of stylistic assessment is individualized instruction which must be designed not to produce conformity or to reduce the divergence of stylistically atypical children in the domain of individual preference and personality. We do not identify uniqueness in order to tag and label children, nor to standardize the modes of thinking that they use and prefer. We are a pluralistic society, and our educational strength lies in an ability not only to tolerate, but to capitalize on that plurality among our children. Therefore, an individualized program of instruction or remediation based on the diagnosis of stylistic nonconformity should continuously take account of the fact that the world of information-processing requires from each of us more than one mode of functioning. We need never deprecate a child's preferred mode of functioning just because we see it as representing a potential deficit in another, often important mode. Rather we must encourage uniqueness; identify classes of academic tasks in which a child's uniqueness is an advantage; teach children how to adopt other strategies for other tasks; and, in the last analysis, teach them to discriminate among tasks and among different approaches to problem solving so that they can both select modes appropriate to the task at hand and select tasks on which their individually preferred mode is most likely to succeed.

REFERENCES

Adams, W.V.: Strategy differences between reflective and impulsive children. *Child Devel, 43*:1076-1080, 1972.

Arner, M.: A Study of Cognitive Style and Its Concomitant Traits and Characteristics in Adolescent Educable Retardates. Unpublished Ph.D. dissertation, New York University, 1973.

Ault, R. L.: Problem-solving strategies of reflective, impulsive, fast-accurate, and slow-inaccurate children. *Child Devel, 44*:259-266, 1973.

Ault, R.L., Crawford, D.E., and Jeffrey, W.E.: Visual scanning strategies of reflective, impulsive, fast-accurate, and slow-inaccurate children on the MFF test. *Child Devel, 43*:1412-1417, 1972.

Baird, R.R., and Bee, H.L.: Modification of conceptual style preference by differential reinforcement. *Child Devel, 40*:903-910, 1969.

Beller, E.K.: Methods of Language Training and Cognitive Styles in Lower-Class Children. Paper presented at American Educational Research Association, New York, February, 1967.

Bjorklund, D.E., and Butter, E.J.: Can impulsivity be predicted from classroom behavior. *J Genet Psychol, 123*:185-194, 1973.

Block, J., Block, J.J., and Harrington, D.M.: Some misgivings about the MFF test as a measure of reflection-impulsivity. *Devel Psychol, 10*:611-632, 1974.

Briggs, C.H.: An Experimental Study of Reflection-Impulsivity in Children. Unpublished Ph.D. dissertation, University of Minnesota, 1966.

Briggs, C.H., and Weinberg, R.A.: Effects of reinforcement in training children's conceptual tempos. *J Ed Psychol, 65*:383-394, 1973.

Broverman, D.M.: Cognitive styles and intra-individual variation in abilities. *J Pers, 28*:240-256, 1960.

Bruner, J.S., Goodnow, J.J., and Austin, G.A.: *A study of thinking.* New York, Wiley, 1966.

Bucky, S.F., Banta, T.J., and Gross, R.B.: Development of motor impulse control and reflectivity. *Percept Mot Skills, 34*:813-814, 1972.

Campbell, S.B.: Mother-child interaction in reflective, impulsive, and hyperactive children. *Devel Psychol, 8*:341-349, 1973.

Campbell, S.B.: Cognitive styles in reflective, impulsive, and hyperactive boys and their mothers. *Percept Mot Skills, 36*:747-752, 1973.

Campbell, S.B., and Douglas, V.I.: Cognitive styles and responses to the threat of frustration. *Can J Beh Sci, 4*:30-42, 1972.

Campbell, S.B., Douglas, V.I., and Morgenstein, G.: Cognitive styles in hyperactive children and the effect of methylphenidate. *J Child Psychol Psychiatry, 12:*55-67, 1971.

Carthcart, G., and Liedtke, W.: Reflectiveness/Impulsiveness and mathematical achievements. *The Arithmetic Teacher, 16:*563-567, 1969.

Chiu, L.H.: Manifest anxiety in children with analytic and nonanalytic cognitive style. *Percept Mot Skills, 35:*406, 1972.

Coates, S.: *Manual for Preschool Embedded Figures Test.* Palo Alto, Consulting Psychologists Press, Inc., 1972.

Constantini, A.F., Corsini, D.A., and Davis, J.E.: Conceptual tempo, inhibition of movement, and acceleration of movement in 4-, 7-, and 9-year old children. *Percept Mot Skills, 37:*779-784, 1973.

Coop, R.: Learning and Cognitive Style: Past, Present, and Future. Paper presented at American Educational Research Association, Los Angeles, 1969.

Coop, R., and Brown, L.: Effects of cognitive style and teaching method on categories of achievement. *J Ed Psychol, 61:*400-405, 1970.

Coop, R.H., and Sigel, I.E.: Cognitive style: Implications for learning and instruction. *Psychology in the Schools, 8:*152-161, 1971.

Davis, A.J.: Cognitive style: Methodological and developmental considerations. *Child Devel, 42:*1447-1459, 1971.

Debus, R.L.: Effect of brief observation of model behavior on conceptual tempo of impulsive children. *Devel Psychol, 2:*22-32, 1970.

Debus, R.L.: A Comparison of Fading, Modeling, and Strategy-Training Techniques for Modifying Conceptual Tempo of Impulsive Children. Unpublished research summary presented at the University of Kansas, September, 1972.

Denmark, F.L., Havelena, R.A., and Murgatroyd, D.: Re-evaluation of some measure of cognitive style. *Percept Mot Skills, 33:*133-134, 1971.

Denney, D.R.: The assessment of differences in conceptual style. *Child Study J, 1:*142-155, 1971.

Denney, D.R.: Modeling effects upon conceptual style and cognitive tempo. *Child Devel, 43:*105-120, 1972a.

Denney, D.R.: Modeling and eliciting effects upon conceptual strategies. *Child Devel, 43:*810-823, 1972b.

Denney, D.R.: Reflection and impulsivity as determinants of conceptual strategy. *Child Devel, 44:*614-623, 1973a.

Denney, D.R.: Modification of children's information processing: A review of the literature. *Child Study Journal Monographs,* (Whole No. 1):1-23, 1973b.

Denney, D.R., and Denney, N.W.: The use of classification for problem solving: A comparison of middle and old age. *Devel Psychol, 9:*275-278, 1973.

Denney, D.R., Denney, N.W., and Ziobrowski, M.J.: Alterations in the information-processing strategies of young children following observation of adult models. *Devel Psychol, 8:*202-208, 1973.

Denney, N.W.: Evidence for Developmental Changes in Categorization Criteria. Unpublished manuscript, University of Kansas, 1973.

Denney, N.W., and Lennon, M.L.: Classification: A comparison of middle and old age. *Devel Psychol, 7:*210-213, 1972.

Drake, D.M.: Perceptual correlates of impulsive and reflective behavior. *Devel Psychol, 2:*202-214, 1970.

Duckworth, S.: The Effects of Selected Visual Discrimination Intervention Conditions on Young Impulsive Retardates. Unpublished Ph.D. dissertation, University of North Carolina, 1972.

Egeland, G.: Training impulsive children in the use of more efficient scanning techniques. *Child Devel, 45:*165-171, 1974.

Errickson, E.A., and Wyne, M.D.: A Response-Cost Procedure for the Reduction of Impulsive Behavior of Academically Handicapped Children. Unpublished manuscript, University of North Carolina, 1972.

Eska, B., and Black, K.N.: Conceptual tempo in young, grade-school children. *Child Devel, 42:*505-516, 1971.

Farley, F., and Farley, S.: Impulsiveness, sociability, and the preference for varied experience. *Percept Mot Skills, 31:*47-50, 1970.

Fleck, J.R.: Cognitive styles in children and performance on Piagetian conservation tasks. *Percept Mot Skills, 35:*747-756, 1972.

Frenkel-Brunswik, E.: Intolerance of ambiguity as an emotional and perceptual personality variable. *J Pers, 18:*108-143, 1949.

Gardner, R.W.: Cognitive Styles in Categorizing Behavior. Unpublished Ph.D. dissertation, University of Kansas, 1952.

Gardner, R.W., Jackson, D.N., and Messick, S.J.: Personality organization in cognitive controls and intellectual abilities. *Psychol Iss,* No. 4:1-140, 1960.

Garrettson, J.: Cognitive style and classification. *J Genet Psychol, 119:*79-87, 1971.

Gorman, B.S., and Wesman, A.E.: The relationship of cognitive style and moods. *J Clin Psychol, 30:*18-25, 1974.

Grieve, T.: The relationship between cognitive style and method of instruction. *J Ed Res, 65:*137-141, 1971.

Grippen, P.C.: Field-independence and reflection-impulsivity as mediators of performance on a programmed learning task with and without strong prompts. *Proceedings of the 81st Annual Convention of the American Psychological Association, Montreal, Canada, 8:*619-620, 1973.

Gruenfeld, L., Weissenberg, P., and Loh, W.: Achievement values, cognitive style and social class: A cross-cultural comparison of Peruvian and U.S. students. *Int J Psychol, 8:*41-49, 1973.

Hallahan, D.P.: Cognitive styles — preschool implications for the disadvantaged. *J Learn Disabil, 3:*7-11, 1970.

Harrison, A., and Nadelman, L.: Conceptual tempo and the inhibition of movement in black preschool children. *Child Devel, 43:*657-668, 1972.

Harsh, J.R.: Cognitive Style—Facilitator or Deterrent to Academic Learning. Claremont Conference on Reading, Claremont, California, 1973.

Heider, E.: Information processing and the modification of an impulsive conceptual tempo. *Child Devel, 42:*1276-1281, 1971.

Hemry, F.P.: Effect of reinforcement conditions on a discrimination learning task for impulsive vs. reflective children. *Child Devel, 44:*657-660, 1973.

Hess, R.D., and Shipman, V.C.: Early experience and the socialization of cognitive modes in children. *Child Devel, 36:*869-886, 1965.

Kagan, J.: Final Progress Report: Passivity and Styles of Thought in Children. Unpublished manuscript, Fels Research Institute, 1964.

Kagan, J.: Individual differences in the resolution of response uncertainty. *J Pers Soc Psychol, 2:*154-160, 1965a.

Kagan, J.: Reflection-impulsivity and reading ability in primary grade children. *Child Devel, 36:*609-628, 1965b.

Kagan, J.: Impulsive and reflective children: Significance of conceptual tempo. In Krumboltz, J.D. (Ed.): *Learning and the Educational Process.* Chicago, Rand, 1965c, pp. 133-161.

Kagan, J.: Body build and conceptual impulsivity in children. *J Pers, 34:* 118-128, 1966a.

Kagan, J.: Developmental studies in reflection and analysis. In Kidd, A.H., and Rivoire, J.H. (Eds.): *Perceptual and Conceptual Development in Children.* New York, Intl Univs Pr, 1966b.

Kagan, J.: Reflection-impulsivity: The generality and dynamics of conceptual tempo. *J Abnorm Psychol, 71:*17-24, 1966c.

Kagan, J.: The role of evaluation in problem solving. In Hellmuth, J. (Ed.): *Cognitive Styles, Vol. 11: Deficits in Cognition.* New York, Brunner-Mazel, 1971.

Kagan, J., and Kogan, N.: Individual variation in cognitive processes. In Mussen, P.H. (Ed.): *Carmichael's Manual of Child Psychology.* New York, Wiley, 1970, Vol. 1, pp. 1273-1365.

Kagan, J., Moss, H.A., and Sigel, I.E.: Psychological significance of styles of conceptualization. In Wright, J.C., and Kagan, J. (Eds.): *Basic Cognitive Processes in Children.* Chicago, U of Chicago Pr, 1973, (First published, *SRCD Monographs,* 1963.)

Kagan, J., Pearson, L., and Welch, L.: Conceptual impulsivity and inductive reasoning. *Child Devel, 37:*583-594, 1966a.

Kagan, J., Pearson, L., and Welch, L.: The modifiability of an impulsive tempo. *J Ed Psychol, 57:*359-365, 1966b.

Kagan, J., and Rossman, B.: Cardiac and respiratory correlates of attention and an analytic attitude. *J Exp Child Psychol, 1:*50-63, 1964.

Kagan, J., Rossman, B., Day, D., Albert, J., and Phillips, W.: Information processing in the child: Significance of analytic and reflective attitudes. *Psychol Monogr, 78,* No. 1, Whole No. 578, 1964.

Katz, J.M.: Reflection-impulsivity and color-form sorting. *Child Devel, 42:* 745-754, 1971.

Katz, J.M.: Cognitive tempo and discrimination skill on color-form sorting tasks. *Percept Mot Skills, 35:*359-362, 1972.

Keogh, B.K.: Psychological evaluation of exceptional children: Old hangups and new directions. *J School Psychol, 10:*141-145, 1972.

Keogh, B.K., and Donlon, G.M.: Field dependence, impulsivity, and learning disabilities. *J Learn Disabil, 5:*331-336, 1972.

Kilburg, R.R., and Siegel, A.W.: Differential feature analysis in the recognition memory of reflective and impulsive children. *Memory and Cognition, 1:*413-419, 1973.

Kling, I.B.: An Experimental Investigation of the Potential of Reflection-Impulsivity as a Determinant of Success in Early Reading Achievement. Unpublished Ph.D. dissertation, Boston College, 1972.

Kogan, N.: Categorizing and Conceptualizing Styles in Younger and Older Children. Research Bulletin (RB-73-66), ETS, Princeton, 1973. ,

Kopfstein, D.: Risk-taking behavior and cognitive styles. *Child Devel, 44:* 190-192, 1973.

Lee, L.C., Kagan, J., and Ralsson, A.: The influence of a preference for analytic categorization upon concept acquisition. *Child Devel, 34:*433-442, 1963.

Lehman, E.B.: Selective strategies in children's attention to task-relevant information. *Child Devel, 43:*197-210, 1972.

Lewis, M., Rausch, M., Goldberg, S., and Dodd, C.: Error, response time and IQ: Sex differences in cognition style of preschool children. *Percept Mot Skills, 26:*563-568, 1968.

Loo, C., and Wenar, C.: Activity level and motor inhibition: Their relation to intelligence test performance in normal children. *Child Devel, 42:*967-971, 1971.

Lowry, P.W., and Ross, L.E.: Severely Retarded Children as Impulsive Responders: Improved Performance With Response Delay. Unpublished manuscript, University of Wisconsin, 1974.

McCluskey, K.A., and Wright, J.C.: Reflection-Impulsivity and Age as Determinants of Visual Scanning Strategy and Preschool Activities. Paper presented at the Society for Research in Child Development, Denver, Colorado, April, 1975.

McCaw, F.: The Relation Between Cognitive Style and Associative Performance in Verbal and Pictorial Concept Formation Tasks. Unpublished manuscript, Indiana University, 1968.

McKinney, J.D.: Developmental study of the acquisition and utilization of conceptual strategies. *J Ed Psychol, 63:*22-31, 1972.

McKinney, J.D.: Problem-solving strategies in impulsive and reflective second graders. *Devel Psychol, 8:*145, 1973.

McKinney, J.D.: "Teacher Perceptions of the Classroom Behavior of Reflec-

240   INTERVENTION WITH HYPERACTIVE CHILDREN

tive and Impulsive Children. Paper presented at Southeastern Physchological Association, 1974.

McKinney, J.D., and Banerjee, C.: Concept Attainment by Reflective and Impulsive Children as a Function of Memory Support. Paper presented at Southeastern Psychological Association, 1974.

Mackworth, N.H.: A stand camera for the line-of-sight recording. *Percept Psychophysics, 2:*119-127, 1967.

Mann, L.: Differences between reflective and impulsive children in tempo and quality of decision making. *Child Devel, 44:*274-279, 1973.

Massari, D., and Massari, J.: Sex differences in the relationship of cognitive style and intellectual functioning in disadvantaged preschool children. *J Genet Psychol, 122:*175-181, 1973.

Massari, D.J., and Schack, M.L.: Discrimination learning by reflective and impulsive children as a function of reinforcement schedule. *Devel Psychol, 6:*183, 1972.

Meichenbaum, D.H.: The Nature and Modification of Impulsive Children: Training Impulsive Children to Talk to Themselves. Research Report, No. 23, Department of Psychology, University of Waterloo, Waterloo, Ontario, Canada, 1971, 1-28. Presented at Society for Research in Child Development, Minneapolis, 1971.

Meichenbaum, D.H., and Goodman, J.: Reflection impulsivity and verbal control of motor behavior. *Child Devel, 40:*785-797, 1969.

Meichenbaum, D.H., and Goodman, J.: Training impulsive children to talk to themselves: A means of developing self-control. *J Abnorm Psychol, 77:* 115-126, 1971.

Messer, S.: The effect of anxiety over intellectual performance on reflection-impulsivity in children. *Child Devel, 41:*723-736, 1970.

Messer, S., and Damarim, F.: Cognitive styles and memory for faces. *J Abnorm Soc Psychol, 69:*313-318, 1964.

Messer, S., and Damarim, F.: Reflection-impulsivity: Stability and school failure. *J Ed Psychol, 61:*487-490, 1970.

Messick, S., and Fritzky, F.J.: Dimensions of analytic attitude in cognition and personality. *J Pers, 31:*346-370, 1963.

Nelson, T.F.: The Effects of Training in Attention Deployment on Observing Behavior in Reflective and Impulsive Children. Unpublished Ph.D. dissertation, University of Minnesota, 1968.

Nuessle, W.: Reflectivity as an influence on focusing behavior of children. *J Exp Child Psychol, 14:*256-276, 1972.

Odom, R.D., McIntyre, C.W., and Neale, G.S.: The influence of cognitive style on perceptual learning. *Child Devel, 42:*883-892, 1971.

Ostfeld, B.M., and Neimark, E.D.: Effect of response time restriction upon cognitive style scores. *Proceedings of the 75th Annual Convention of the American Psychological Association, 2:*169-170, 1967.

Palkes, H., Stewart, M., and Kahana, B.: Porteus maze performance of hyperactive boys after training in self-directed verbal commands. *Child Devel, 39:*817-826, 1968.

Reali, N., and Hall, V.: Effects of success and failure on the reflective and impulsive child. *Devel Psychol, 3:*392-402, 1970.

Reppucci, N.D.: Antecedents of Conceptual Tempo in the Two-Year-Old Child. Unpublished Ph.D. dissertation, Harvard University, 1968.

Reppucci, N.D.: Individual Differences in the Consideration of Information Among Two-Year-Old Children. *Devel Psychol, 2:*240-246, 1970.

Ridberg, E.H., Parke, R.D., and Hetherington, E.M.: Modification of impulsive and reflective cognitive styles through observation of film-mediated models. *Devel Psychol, 5:*369-377, 1971.

Rosman, B.L.: Analytic Cognitive Style in Children. Unpublished Ph.D. dissertation, Yale University, 1962.

Ruble, D.N., and Nakamura, C.Y.: Task orientation vs. social orientation in young children and their attention to relevant social cues. *Child Devel, 43:*471-480, 1972.

Salkind, N.J., and Wright, J.C.: Reflection-Impulsivity and Cognitive Efficiency: An Integrated Model. 1975 (in preparation).

Santostefano, S., Rutledge, L., and Randall, D.: Cognitive styles and reading disability. *Psychol in the Schools, 2:*57-62, 1965.

Schack, M.L., and Massari, D.J.: The Effect of Conceptual Tempo and Reinforcement Conditions on Probability Learning. Paper presented at Biennial Meeting of the Society for Research in Child Development, Minneapolis, April, 1971.

Scher, S.S.: The Effects of Fading, Reinforcement, or Withdrawal of Reinforcement on Impulsive Responding. Unpublished master's thesis, C.W. Post College, Long Island University, 1971.

Schwebel, A.I.: Effects of impulsivity on performance of verbal tasks in middle and lower-class children. *Am J Orthopsychiatry, 36:*13-21, 1966.

Schwebel, A.I., and Bernstein, A.J.: The effects of impulsivity on the performance of lower-class children on form WISC subtests. *Am J Orthopsychiatry, 40:*629-636, 1970.

Scott, N., and Sigel, I.E.: Effects of Inquiry Training in Physical Science on Creativity and Cognitive Styles of Elementary School Children. Research report for USOE, 1965.

Shine, N.: Cognitive impulsivity and Piaget's theory of perceptual decentration. *Dissertation Abstracts International, 32-B:*2385-2386, 1971.

Siegel, A.W., Kirasic, K.C., and Kilburg, R.R.: Recognition memory in reflective and impulsive preschool children. *Child Devel, 44:*651-656, 1973.

Sigel, I.E.: Styles of Categorization in Elementary School Children: The Role of Sex Differences and Anxiety Level. Paper presented at the meeting of the Society for Research in Child Development, Minneapolis, March, 1965.

Sigel, I.E., Jarman, P., and Hanesian, H.: Styles of categorization and their intellectual and personality correlates in young children. *Human Devel, 10*:1-17, 1967.

Siegelman, E.Y.: Reflective and impulsive observing behavior. *Child Devel, 40*:1213-1222, 1969.

Singer, S., and Smith, I.L.: Assessment of Reflectivity-Impulsivity in Primary Level Educable Mentally Retarded Children. Paper presented at American Educational Research Association, Chicago, 1974.

Spotts, J.V., and Mackler, B.: Relationships of Field-Dependent and Field-Independent Cognitive Styles to Creative Test Performance. *Percept Mot Skills, 24*:239-268, 1967.

Stanes, D., and Gordon, A.: Relationships between CST and children's EFT. *J Pers, 41*:185-191, 1973.

Stevens, D.A., Boydstun, J.A., Ackerman, P.T., and Dykman, R.A.: Reaction time, impulsivity, and autonomic lability in children with minimal brain dysfunction. *Proceedings of the 76th Annual Convention of the American Psychological Association,* 1968.

Strommen, E.: Verbal self-regulation in a children's game: Impulsive errors on "Simon Says". *Child Devel, 44*:849-853, 1973.

Sutton-Smith, B., and Rosenberg, B.G.: A scale to identify impulsive behavior in children. *J Genet Psychol, 95*:211-216, 1959.

Sutton-Smith, B., and Rosenberg, B.G.: Impulsivity and sex preference. *J Genet Psychol, 98*:187-192, 1961.

Sykes, D.H., Douglas, V.I., Weiss, G., and Minde, K.K.: Attention in hyperactive children and the effect of methylphenidate (Ritalin). *J Child Psychol Psychiatry, 12*:129-139, 1971.

Vleitstra, A.G., and Wright, J.C.: The Effect of Strategy Training, Stimulus Saliency, and Age on Recognition in Preschoolers. Unpublished Ph.D. dissertation, University of Kansas, 1973 and Progress Report, Kansas Center for Research in Early Childhood Education, September, 1973.

Vurpillot, E.: The development of scanning strategies and their relation to visual discrimination. *J Exp Child Psychol, 6*:632-650, 1968.

Ward, W.C.: Creativity in young children. *Child Devel, 39*:737-754, 1968a.

Ward, W.C.: Reflection-impulsivity in kindergarten children. *Child Devel, 39*:867-874, 1968b.

Weinberg, R.A.: The Effects of Different Types of Reinforcement in Training a Reflective Conceptual Tempo. Unpublished Ph.D. dissertation, University of Minnesota. Ann Arbor, Michigan: University Microfilms, 1969, No. 69, 1560.

Weir, M.W.: Developmental changes in problem solving strategies. *Psychol Rev, 71*:473-490, 1964.

Welch, L.: A Naturalistic Study of Free Play Behavior of Reflective and Impulsive Four-Year-Olds. Presented at the Society for Research in Child Development, Philadelphia, 1973.

Werner, H.: *Comparative Psychology of Mental Development*, 2nd Ed. New York, Science Editions, 1961.

White, S.H.: Evidence for a hierarchical arrangement of learning processes. In Lipsitt, L.P., and Spiker, C.C. (Eds.): *Advances in Child Development and Behavior*. New York, Academic, 1965, 2, 187-220.

Witkin, H.A.: Origins of cognitive style. In Sheerer, C, (Ed.): *Cognition, theory, research, promise*. New York, Harper Row, 1964, pp. 172-205.

Wright, J.C.: Reflection-Impulsivity and Associated Observing Behaviors in Preschool Children. Paper presented at the Society for Research in Child Development, Minneapolis, 1971a.

Wright, J.C.: *The Kansas Reflection-Impulsivity Scale for Preschoolers*. (KRISP). St. Louis, CEMREL, 1971b.

Wright, J.C.: The KRISP: A Technical Report. Annual Report, Kansas Center for Research in Early Childhood Education, 1972.

Wright, J.C.: *A User's Manual for the KRISP*. St. Louis, CEMREL, 1973.

Wright, J.C.: Reflection-Impulsivity and Information Processing from Three to Nine Years of Age. Paper presented at the American Psychological Association meetings, New Orleans, 1974.

Wright, J.C., and Vlietstra, A.G.: The development of selective attention: From perceptual exploration to logical search. In Reese, H. (Ed.): *Advances in Child Development and Behavior*. New York, Academic Press, in press, vol. 10.

Wolfe, R., Egelston, R., and Powers, J.: Conceptual structure and conceptual tempo. *Percept Mot Skills, 35*:331-337, 1972.

Yando, R.M., and Kagan, J.: The effect of teacher tempo on the child. *Child Devel, 39*:27-34, 1968.

Yando, R.M., and Kagan, J.: The effect of task complexity on reflection-impulsivity. *Cognitive Psychol, 1*:192-220, 1970.

Yeatts, P.P., and Strag, G.A.: Flexibility of cognitive style and its relationship to academic achievement in 4th and 6th grades. *J Ed Res, 64*:345-346, 1971.

Zelniker, T., Jeffrey, W.E., Ault, R., and Parsons, J.: Analysis and modification of search strategies for impulsive and reflective children on the Matching Familiar Figures Test. *Child Devel, 43*:321-335, 1972.

Zelniker, T., and Oppenheimer, L.: Modification of information processing of impulsive children. *Child Devel, 44*:445-450, 1973.

Zucker, J.S., and Stricker, G.: Impulsivity-reflectively in preschool headstart and middle-class children. *J Learn Disabil, 1*:578-584, 1968.

7

The measurement of
hyperactivity: trends and issues
Neil J. Salkind and John P. Poggio

A REVIEW OF THE LITERATURE suggests that the teacher, psychologist or pediatrician would search far and wide in their respective fields before discovering a classification term more frequently employed than *hyperactivity* to describe a syndrome of disruptive behaviors. The majority of descriptions are vague and nonoperational, and just as frequently the techniques used in the assessment of the syndrome fall short of providing documentary evidence relative to the validity of the measurement or evaluative procedure. Searching through the literature it is apparent that a premium has been placed on the results of assessment techniques rather than how the limitations of such techniques might affect subsequent intervention and treatment. Although conceptual definitions are necessary when formulating a theoretical perspective, it is the operational definition that the practitioner must deal with in his research or treatment program. Furthermore, the relative ease with which hyperactivity has been "operationally" defined presents a background against which results of reported research are ambiguous, unclear, nonspecific, inconclusive and frequently lack generalizability, thus making replication almost impossible.

Such cited symptoms as overactivity, distractibility, impulsiveness, excitability and no less than twenty remaining descriptors have been generously applied in an attempt to describe what characterizes the syndrome. Such a state of affairs leaves the researcher and the practitioner holding an elaborately decorated but somewhat empty bag. This degree of imprecision can undoubtedly place the child in the mistaken position of being subjected to well-intentioned but inaccurate diagnosis and treatment. What appears to be a fundamental difficulty in the assessment of hyperactivity, then, is that procedures are not adequately documented from the perspective of construct validity, and they too frequently differ from researcher to researcher even when identical hypotheses are being investigated. The purposes of this chapter are (1) to present a survey of the pertinent issues involved in the assessment of hyperactivity, (2) to review some of the existing methods employed in the measurement and evaluation of activity level and/or hyperactivity in children, and (3) to present a model which synthesizes the methodological concerns and limitations inherent within the research that has been completed.

THEORETICAL ISSUES

An extensive review by Cromwell, Baumeister and Hawkins (1963) on the definition, measurement of and theoretical approaches towards the general area of activity level established guidelines and formulated questions that are germane to any discussion of hyperactivity. These authors described four methods of measuring activity level: direct visual observation, free space traversal, figeometric and kinometric, as well as noting the distinguishing features amongst them. They point out how different techniques for assessment may be ignoring important intraindividual characteristics highly related to the type of activity being measured regardless of the method being employed. For example, where direct visual observation may consider the frequency of a behavior to be the factor that best identifies the behavior, a fidgeometric technique such as the ballistograph measures the degree (intensity) to which the subject jars or vibrates the platform on which he is placed. In this case, although frequency and intensity might be relatively independent of each other, they both indicate that activity is taking place. At this time there is an absence of consistent evidence.

To illustrate, McConnell and Cromwell (1964) discuss activity level as the lower limit or lower bound of hyperactivity, yet their comparison between scores on the Child Rating Scale (CRS), which includes those behavioral terms most often used in describing the syndrome, and the ballistograph found the two to be unrelated to each other. Schulman, Kasper and Throne (1965) also failed to find a statistically significant relationship between total activity as measured by the actometer and some other behavioral indices they examined. Yet discrepancies do not just exist across different methodologies in assessment. For example, Conrad and Dusell (1967) documented a discrepancy between the experimental claim of positive results and clinical impressions by practitioners in the effectiveness of amphetamines. Further complicating this lack of clarity are findings such as those of Schulman et al. (1965) who observed normal children exhibiting a wide range of activity level with the standard deviation frequently exceeding the magnitude of the arithmetic mean.

The absence of relationships between various methods for assessing hyperactivity has not entirely been the case. Foshbee (1958), in measuring hyperactivity, found the correlation between a mechanical device (the ballistograph) and outside judges using stop watch techniques to be 0.89. Victor, Halverson and Buczkowski (1973) found a substantial correlation (r = 0.77) between teachers' ratings and ratings derived from an activity recorder. Halverson and Waldrop (1973) also found a statistically significant correlation (r = 0.51) between the use of the activity recorder and teachers' ratings.

Explanations of the discrepancies noted above might be attributed to (1) the existence of more than one type of activity level or form of hyperactivity, and/or (2) the use of measurement instruments (procedures) that are unreliable and lack validity across situations or subjects. Investigations need to be undertaken that would clarify the important questions of how many types/ kinds of activity levels do exist and how these types differ from each other both qualitatively and quantitatively.

Cromwell et al. (1963), in summarizing earlier research, points out that "information available is sufficient to suggest that activity level should not be viewed as a single or homogenous phenomenon (p. 365)." Reed (1947) earlier expressed similar thoughts in writing "what data we have, points to more than one type, or at least more than one aspect of activity (p. 305)." In support of such claims, Morgan and Stellar (1950) specified three bipolar descriptors of activity level—locomotor versus diffuse, relevant versus irrelevant and goal—directed versus nongoal-directed. Loo and Wenar more recently (1971) have delineated three types of activity— activity level as the quantitative amount of notoric movements, motor inhibition as the degree of ability to inhibit motor impulses, and impulsivity as the lack of self-control in modes other than motoric. Interestingly, the last pair of polarities that Morgan and Stellar identify have more recently been used as discriminators between hyperactive and nonhyperactive children (Bell, Waldrop, and Weller, 1972). In the development of a movement recording device, Bell (1968) has concluded that there exists more than one type of activity, and that "components and manifestations of activity in different measurement situations should be studied rather than activity as a unitary invariant function (p. 303). Differences in motoric activity have been interpreted by Campbell (1968) as an indicator of the impact of the environment, situation or conditions which influence the infant's response to stimulation, or as an innate or genetic feature of a child's behavior. Pope and Pope (1969) raise the issue that a number of different levels or types of activity are of importance, and that any attempt at defining hyperactivity should take into account both the amount of activity as well as the focus and direction. Similarly, Cromwell et al. (1963) indicated the "superactivity" may be illusory or unreal because of the short attention span and frequent shifts in goal direction—that is, estimates of another individual's activity level are often interpreted in light of a variety of interrelated factors. These studies appear to allow the following conclusions: activity level itself has been conceptualized in numerous ways, and a number of different types or levels of activity have been identified. The result has been that different techniques and instruments have focused on subclasses or categories of activity level. Aside from being alarming to the interested observer, the impact would appear to be greater confusion, inconsistent findings and a fragmented view of the behavior by individuals embracing their own definition and assessment methodology. It would appear that an effort to create a taxonomy of activity level would indeed be a purposeful venture. Such a taxonomy would allow the classification of different types of activity levels, modes of hyperactivity and other relevant behaviors to provide a more clearly-defined conceptual base from which fundamental "conclusions" as those mentioned earlier might be further investigated.

A fundamental difficulty encountered in the study of activity level is that standards (norms) for what constitutes *normal* (acceptable) activity level(s) do not exist. All too often a standard is left to the subjective interpretation of a definition or a description of a behavior which is enveloped in clinical terms. Such a shortcoming is common among those instruments that employ observer's judgments. It is conceivable that the absence of operational norms could result in a discrete classification of a sample of children (all of whom are quite *normal* relative to the behavior hyperactivity) as hyperactive, normal and hypoactive. Schmitt, Martin, Nellhaus, Cravens, Camp and Jordan (1973) imply some normative structure by defining a hyperactive child as one whose motor activity is excessive for someone of his mental age and sex. Excessive activity is said to exist when several people complain about it. While this is a start, it is hardly sufficient, and there does exist the need for quantitatively established norms that allow researchers and/or practitioners to identify the limits and extremes of activity.

The danger in defining hyperactivity without the benefit of a sound empirical base is that the definition and specification of different types of activity will have a direct influence on the measurement and evaluation procedures used or developed to assess the behaviors. The most popular practice and perhaps the one most lacking in construct validity is the assignment of synonyms that reflect behaviors similar to those descriptive of the hyperactive child, but do not broaden or advance the validity of any definition. Keogh (1971) has commented that "most investigators focus on the symptomatology of the condition without defining the construct."

Adding confusion to an already-nebulous issue, the term *hyperkinetic* has been a derivative of or used as a synonym for such terms as *hyperactive, overactivity, hypermotility neurosis, minimal brain dysfunction, postencephaltic behavior disorder* and *organic driveness.* Such terminology is not meant to be synonomous in either etiology or recommended treatment, but it does increase the difficulty of valid assessment. In fact these terms often subsume themselves. For example, hyperactivity is stated by Clements (1966) as being one of the ten most often cited characteristics of minimal brain dysfunction. Aronson (1971) also questions whether the hyperkinetic syndrome is an underlying factor related to minimal brain dysfunction. Although a rose by any other name is still a rose, procedural differences should deal directly with the critical question being asked, in this case "What constitutes hyperactivity?" Different terminologies and theoretical orientations do indeed lend themselves to different measurement procedures. Similarly, a set of one-word descriptors having at best only content or face validity are frequently used to describe the syndrome, making diagnosis an easier but far less exact task. It should be understood that when a label is employed to describe a set of behaviors which intuitively appear to be related, the conditions and limitations of such a label must also be presented. Other terms offered as descriptive of the hyperactive child and indicative of some behavioral components of the syndrome itself are short attention span, mood fluctuation, impulsivity, restlessness and distractibility. A content analysis of the research done in the area of hyperactivity would yield interesting results as to the overlap and frequency of the same descriptors which appear.

Empirical evidence has been offered that questions the validity of such descriptors. For example, Werry (1968) has found no reliable data demonstrating that hyperactive children have an attentional deficit (short attention span) as measured by the WISC coding subtest. Interestingly, terminology that is equally characteristic and descriptive of other childhood difficulties is also frequently employed in describing the hyperactive child; examples include negativism, poor judgment and irritability (Delong, 1972). In sum, assigning descriptive and operationally valid terms is a necessary input for guiding the evaluation process.

Attempts have been made to define hyperactivity as a function of a specific setting. Zrull, Westman, Arthur and Rice (1966) cited research that indicates children who are judged to be "clinically hyperactive" do not display more gross activity per day than normal children, and what is judged as hyperactive may not be due to total activity but to a failure to inhibit motor activity when appropriate. Buddenhagen and Seehler (1969) contend that hyperactivity describes those aspects of a person's behavior which annoy the observer. Werry (1968) defines hyperactivity as "a chronic, sustained, excessive level of motor activity which is the cause of significant and continued complaint both at home and at school (p. 171)." Similarly, Battle and Lacey (1972) define hyperactivity as "the degree to which the subject's motor behavior was described in home visits, nursery school, and day camps as impulsive, uninhibited, and uncontrolled. . . .(p. 760)." Coincidentally, these authors then assessed hyperactivity using a device that monitored arm and leg movements during periods of data gathering. What these definitions share in common is an effort to describe hyperactivity within the context which the behavior occurs. This effort is unfortunately defeated by the resultant lack of generalizability across situations as well as children. The role of the stimuli in the situation where activity is being measured is critically important since changes in activity level may in fact be a function of the stimulus control. The research literature that focuses on basic learning theory, especially S-R theory, regards both stimulus *and* reinforcement control as powerful determinants of behavior. For example, the incidence of hyperactivity is so high in certain settings that it is assumed the child suffers from the syndrome simply because this is the most frequently occurring cluster of "behavior problems" in the classroom from a probabilistic point of view (Kenny, Clemens, Hudson, Leutz, Cicci, and Nair, 1971).

Some investigators have studied hyperactivity as a categorical or independent variable for including or excluding a child from a population to be studied in research on motor activity. For a child to be labelled as hyperactive in one such study, overactivity had to be the major complaint by both parents (home setting) and teachers (school setting) (Sykes, Douglas, Weiss, and Minde, 1971). An extreme case of a situation-specific definition of hyperactivity is illustrated by Routh and Roberts (1972). They examined covariation among selected behavioral deviations descriptive of the minimal brain dysfunction syndrome and considered the child hyperactive if "the clinic staff unanimously judged him to be either overactive or severely hyperkinetic on the day of evaluation, or if he was currently on medication" (p. 308) or "if his teacher checked the terms overactive (severe) as applying to the child on the school protocol (p. 309)." It is apparent in such a case that a disproportionate amount of dependency on external criteria or personal definitions overrides and prevents the formation of a consistent operational approach to definition. The writers' earlier comments relating to the need for norms and standards seem germane at this point when seeking a solution to the problem of accurate classification.

In sum, there appears to be a widespread practice of defining and operating within the sphere of the hyperactive child using techniques and/or instruments that often lack a substantial degree of validity. The task, then, is to subdivide component parts of the concept hyperactivity into more manageable and testable units relating both definitional and assessment procedures to one another. Although the intuitive approach so often taken is sometimes revealed as proper, it is the lack of generalizability, and control that severely limits and negates these efforts. Assessment in itself cannot function independently of definition, just as the definitional process cannot be viewed as being independent of the etiology and theoretical basis for hyperactivity. In order to more clearly represent the relationship between the measurement technique employed (assessment procedure) and the theoretical orientation to the syndrome entitled *hyperactivity*, a two-dimensional matrix will be presented. Four classifications as outgrowths of theoretical approaches to hyperactivity serve as one dimension of this two-dimensional matrix while the nature of the assessment technique employed characterizes the second.

CLASSIFICATION OF RESEARCH

In an attempt to more fully elaborate upon the relationship between the theoretical basis of the construct hyperactivity (implicitly or explicitly expressed) and the method of assessment employed, a two-dimensional figure is presented below. The intersections between these dimensions, e.g. developmental/checklist, are a major consideration when evaluating the status of hyperactivity as a construct. It should be noted that any one level of a dimension is not necessarily of equal importance across all levels of the other dimension. For example, one theoretical definition might very effectively be suited to a specific assessment technique but not very well suited to the other assessment techniques. Such an interactive matrix should enable the reader to more clearly define immediate goals and objectives in a program focussing on hy-

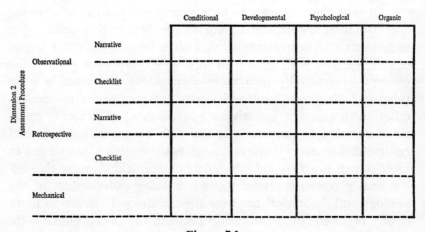

Figure 7-1.

peractive children since both method and theory are addressed simultaneously.

The following section of this paper further discusses each of these dimensions by treating each level individually and focussing on the relationship between the levels of the dimensions and the construct of hyperactivity.

Dimension 1: The Assumed Basis for the Theoretical Definition of the Construct

The theoretical definition of the construct refers to the nature of causal factors involved in documenting the syndrome. This dimension consists of four classifications—*conditional, developmental, psychological* and *organic*—under which behaviors categorized as hyperactive reflect the different orientations taken toward the syndrome. Schmidt (1974) presented four similar categories accompanied by a brief symptomology of each category that were meant to be diagnostic. Unlike Schmidt's scheme, these classifications have been employed as indicators of the theoretical assumptions inherent within the definition assumed. Just as any syndrome might consist of a variety of behaviors, each classification should not be thought of as being necessarily independent and/or mutually exclusive of the others.

Theoretical Definition 1: Conditional

The first category is defined as a syndrome of activities resulting primarily from a set of external factors that maintain and/or control behaviors characterized as hyperactive and possibly are precluded by some developmental and/or genetic component. Such a definitional approach might accurately reflect the theoretical position assumed by a social learning theorist or a behaviorist who contends that patterns of behavior are acquired which conform to social expectations, and are appropriately reinforced, e.g. operant conditioning. Observational learning as a result of modeling and imitation are characteristic of this classification. An example of such a theoretical orientation is found in the research of Battle and Lacey (1972). As noted earlier, Battle and Lacey defined hyperactivity as the degree of motor activity in specific settings or conditions (home, nursery school and day camp). The behavior is considered to be conditional (or contingent) on a variety of factors, e.g. parental attention, teacher behaviors, peer group relationships, sibling rivalry behavioral settings and other influences external to the child. Kenny et al. (1971) illustrated how hyperactive children can demonstrate levels of motor activity which were appropriate depending upon the environment, and that environmental factors may be a class of events that when interacting with certain biological elements result in hyperactive behavior. At present little research has been conducted outside of those single subject designs yielding information as to the specific factors responsible for hyperactivity. For those studies conducted, factors for which *hyperactive behaviors* were found to be contingent have been operationally specified and shown to be highly individualized and situation specific. Therefore, it is difficult to conclude that a set of factors exists across all situations. Appropriate synonyms for the classification *conditional* would be exogenous, circumstantial, situational, environmental, cultural, extrinsic and social.

Theoretical Definition 2: Developmental

The second definitional category is termed *developmental*. It is proposed to identify a syndrome of activities based on a predisposition toward behavior(s) characterized as hyperactive that are transmitted through genetic mechanisms and are possibly elicited by some situational or environmental condition. Werry (1968) found evidence for a degree of developmental predisposition towards hyperactivity in that 64 percent of the families he examined had histories of similar pathological disturbances. Morrison and Stewart (1971) have noted that relatives of hyperactive children have a high occurrence of psychiatric illness, most frequently alcoholism, but with an excess of hysteria and sociopathy. They conclude that hyperactivity may be a childhood prologue to alcoholism and other behavioral disorders and conclude that "regardless of the nature of transmission, our data indicate the association of a specific childhood problem with a specific disorder in the parents." Cantwell (1972) attempted to characterize a parent as having been a hyperactive child and found a high percentage of the parents of hyperactive children were psychiatrically ill themselves. Further evidence for a developmental component is offered by Willerman (1973) who has presented evidence to show that strong associations exist between the activity level of parents and the activity levels of their children (which can be interpreted as conditional as well). The theoretical classification *developmental* supports the viewpoint that hyperactivity is primarily a disorder that is transmitted genetically.

Theoretical Definition 3: Psychological

The third definitional category, identified as *psychological,* is viewed as a syndrome of activities originating from psychological processes used in dealing with the world in an everyday sense and resulting in behavior classified as hyperactive. The underlying assumption of such a theoretical viewpoint is that hyperactive behavior is the result of defective or ineffective psychological systems which are impaired to such an extent that the individual is prevented from meeting the ordinary demands of everyday life. As the case with the theoretical classification *conditional,* the presence of ineffective psychological processes is highly individualized. Whether it be a lack of ego resilience or ego strength, the resultant behavior is difficult to define and treat due to the abstract nature of the etiology. A good illustration of such a theoretical position is the "hydraulic energy" and other psychoanalytic theories that postulate the need to discharge pent-up energies. Within this model an example of a deficient system from which hyperactivity would result might be faulty ego development and the resultant lack of impulse control. Such functional abnormalities when not accompanied by some clearly organic or developmental component are extremely difficult to operationally defined and measure. Other terms used to denote a similar category might be *functional* or *psychogenic.*

Theoretical Definition 4: Organic

Lastly, the categorization *organic* is defined as that syndrome of activities resulting from a demonstratable abnormality in the structure and/or biochemistry of bodily tissues and/or organs. Laufer, Denhoff and Solomons (1957) have suggested that the syndrome results from an injury or dysfunction of the diencehphalon in early life. The result of this condition is an extreme sensitivity (of the central nervous system) to stimuli constantly bombarding peripheral receptors. While the hypothesis of some organic dysfunction is highly tenable, certain methodological problems in studying such causal factors have been enumerated by Chalfant and Schifflen (1969).

The condition of hyperactivity is not easily identified as being caused by organic dysfunctions when an extensive period of time has passed between the onset of the original disorder and eventual postmortem examination. Second, there exists a lack of adequate methods for the examination of brain functioning when gross neurological damage is not immediately apparent. Third, although the behavioral abnormality may be fully accounted for by some organic disorder, the lack of sensitive instruments tends to inhibit purposeful research in identifying causal factors.

When the syndrome was first described by Ingram (1956) most clinicians assumed it to be the result of brain damage, but the last few years have yielded information that only a small percentage of children having a history of hyperactivity are indeed brain damaged (Chess, 1959; Stewart, Pitts, Craig, and Dieruf, 1966; and Minde et al., 1968). Kenny et al. (1971) have concluded that the use of extensive medical examinations to identify the hyperactive child appears "relatively unrewarding." Clemmens and Kenny (1972) reported that the need for neurological examination prior to placement in special education programs is inappropriate. This category, *organic,* can also be referred to as morphological.

The syndrome characterized by hyperactive behavior(s) is by no means a clearly identifiable pattern from a diagnostic or causal perspective. The research questions that yet need to be answered are "What is the nature of the underlying communalities across these four classifications? and "What are the unique elements within each classification that contribute to a robust definition?" To the practitioner the four classifications presented should be seen as mutually interdependent and, thus, in any complete examination of factors involved in the determination of hyperactivity, consideration of each of these categories is essential.

Dimension 2: Assessment Procedure

The second dimension of the classificatory scheme, the assessment procedure, refers to the methodology by which the behavior is being evaluated and not the behavior per se. For example, although a mechanical instrument might be used to assess hyperactivity, the primary concern in this dimension is the applicability and appropriateness of the instrument, not the cause, intensity or duration of the behavior being measured. This dimension has been divided into three methodological categories—observational assessment, retrospective assessment and mechanical assessment. Each procedure will be described, and examples of research where such techniques were applied will be discussed.

Assessment Procedure 1: Observational

Observational assessment procedures consist of the observing and recording of events by trained observers such that the behavior occurring is recorded within the stream of natural occurrence. In common among these procedures is the fact that the behavior is recorded at the time of occurrence or very shortly thereafter. An example of these procedures might be time and point sampling which are applicable when the data is recorded concurrently with or shortly following the observation. Time and point sampling are techniques where samples of behavior are selected either systematically or at random in order to be representative of a population of behavioral units larger than those observed during the sample. Examples of such assessment procedures might be behavorial checklists and record charts. An issue often encountered, yet only superficially addressed is that of the reliability of such observational techniques. As reliability is a neccessary, yet not a sufficient condition for validity, this characteristic of a measurement device or assessment technique should be considered as a major component of any evaluative process. Reliability can most easily be conceptualized as the relationship between true or errorless score plus any error which might enter into the assessment itself.

Examples of potential sources of error might be situational variables, lack of standardization, etc. Relating more closely to the present discussion, examples of such errors are the use of untrained observers, or mechanical instruments that have not been properly calibrated. The higher this error in relation to the true score, the lower the reliability. Typically, observational procedures have lower reliabilities than mechanical or even self-report instruments due to their susceptibility to human error but lend themselves to a much broader range in type and quality of observation and subsequent interpretation.

Laufer et al. (1957) attempted to provide a reliable set of descriptors to be used by observers when assessing the syndrome they entitled "hyperkinetic impulse disorder." Such an early effort should be applauded as an attempt at operationalizing definitions. For example, the meaning of the description *irritability* is depicted as a low frustration tolerance. Admittedly, the same difficulties in evaluation arise in assigning an empirically sound referent to low frustration tolerance as to irritability, but a first step in the proposed direction was attempted.

Rating scales are also frequently employed to assess hyperactivity. A rating is a judgment along some predefined continuum where the teacher (observer) is required to rate a child from high to low on a variety of characteristics. McConnell and Cromwell (1964) employed the Child Rating Scale (CRS) mentioned earlier. In their study attendants who received training in the use of the scale were asked to rate the behavior of each child "as observed by you over the past three days." The test-retest reliability per rater for this exercise averaged 0.84. Connors (1969) employed a behavior rating scale in describing five behavioral factors. Hyperactivity was the fourth factor and was characterized by behaviors such as sitting and fiddling with small objects, humming and making other noises, excitability and teasing other children. Bell, Waldrop and Weller (1972) used teachers' and parents' ratings on a behavior assessment system that measures extremes of hyperactive behavior. The results of these ratings were the creation of six scales which were frenetic play, induction of intervention, nomadic play, spilling and throwing, inability to delay, and emotional aggression.

While the scale has been developed, there has yet to be reported any evidence of cross validation.

Other observational procedures employ special conditions. For example, Hutt (1963) used a room with grids marked on the floor to measure duration and location of movement. Similarly, Cromwell et al. (1963) describe studies where the subject is free and unrestricted, and where, for example, the floor is marked into grids as *free space traversal*. Halverson and Waldrop (1973) recorded cumulative time spent in various indoor activities using frequency counts. Observer reliability was found to exceed 0.90. In the same study, daily rating summaries by teachers were also employed on an eleven-point scale with resulting high interrater reliability (r = 0.88). Victor, Halverson and Buczkowski (1973), in a comparison of observational and mechanical techniques, employed a checklist of behavioral referents and the number of floor squares traversed. The behavioral referents listed are similar to those listed by Bell et al. (1972), e.g. teases, annoys, jumps around excessively, and is overexcited. General observational techniques may take the form of narratives where, for example, specimen records or ecological descriptions and other narrative types of data would be collected (Wright, 1960). Observational methods might also include such procedures as checklists where data is recorded as a reflection of the existence or nonexistence of specific categories or classes of behavior. One such example is the CRS employed by McConnell and Cromwell (1964).

In general, observational techniques as those identified above are simple to perform and require a minimum amount of equipment. Two disadvantages of these techniques, however, are the need for a full-time observer and the high probability of human error (subjectivity) entering into the measurement process. In their discussion of an underlying mechanism being responsible for hyperactivity, Laufer et al. (1957) comment how history is an extremely valuable tool in diagnosis.

Assessment Procedure 2: Retrospective

The second class of assessment procedures is termed *retrospective* assessment techniques. Retrospective assessment techniques are those wherein the respondent is asked to recall certain events or characteristics such as previous activity levels, familial psychological disturbances, medical history, etc. Narrative and checklist procedures are appropriate as well when using a retrospective methodology. The distinction between narrative and checklist is the structure of the stimulus used to elicit information. Where narrative retrospective methods employ relatively open-ended questions, retrospective checklists are highly structured and impose restrictions on the subject's response.

Narrative types of assessment techniques are employed where behavioral events are reproduced in the same sequence as their original occurrence, e.g. the recalling of family relationships over an extended period of time and/or feelings toward selected members. Checklist devices are also convenient for obtaining information since they employ a variety of categories and can be conveniently employed. While the checklist format provides categories of behavior, the richness and detail that arises from the use of anecdotes, for example a narrative technique, can often be more informative. The choice of technique does depend upon a host of situational variables such as location, time constraints, purpose of observation and impact of the technique on the target behavior. The vast majority of research that has hypothesized a relationship between the hyperactivity of the child and some familial characteristics, e.g. Morrison and Stewart (1971), employ a form of interview or checklist that in part requires information about behavior or incidents that have occurred at some prior time. The finding of Howell (1972) that parents of hyperactive children remember their child having feeding and sleeping problems in the first year of life (significantly more so than normal children) required parents to retrieve information not readily available in a temporal sense. This example effectively illustrates such a retrospective technique. This class of procedures then enables the investigator to survey previously unavailable sources of information keeping in perspective that such information is often biased and situation specific in nature. What often occurs is the creation of a series of different techniques which are then employed independently of theoretical rationale. This is by no means the case for all such attempts at assessment, but there is a large proportion of literature for which this mutual interdependency between theory and method is lacking.

Assessment Procedure 3: Mechanical

The final category of assessment procedures is *mechanical,* where data is collected employing some type of a mechanical device. These techniques do not suffer from the threat of human variability in judging behavior, but are rigid in their application and frequently prohibitively expensive and inconvenient for the subject.

Under the classification of mechanical methods of evaluating activity/hyperactivity, Cromwell et al. (1963) specify two classes of mechanical procedures—kinometric and fidgeometric. For example, the kinometric approach consists of attaching to the individual a single or a series of instruments such as the actometer (a modified set of wristwatches placed to record activity in the three planes of movement—up/down, left/right, forward/backward). The pedometer is another example. Schulman and Reisman (1959) introduced this modified wrist watch worn by the child (on the wrist) in order to record behavior. Bell (1968) later developed a smaller and less expensive model measuring the number of movements a subject might make. Johnson (1971), after examining the reliability of the actometer, criticizes its use as being "dramatically unequally sensitive to all movement." Further, he states the actometer is "not reliable, and the relationship of the motion they qualitate to the behavior of the hyperactive child would be questionable." In a study by Kaspar and Lowenstein (1971) the actometer was used, but the authors feel it important to consider the antecedent activity level of the subjects and to preserve that prior to the measurement session. Loo and Wenar (1971) also employed the actometer to differentiate the three types of behavior mentioned earlier. In this study, impulsiveness, although a commonly used descriptor of hyperactive children, was found not to correlate with their assessment of hyperactivity. Maccoby, Powley, Hagan and Degerman (1965) also found that the test-retest reliability for the actometer is higher for girls than

for boys. Pope (1970) has used an instrument similar to the actometer (the accelerometer) attached to the wrist of the writing hand
and to the ankle on the same side. The measure of activity is a
combination of the two readings. Combining two such scores to
form a single linear composite could possibly confound the final
interpretation of the data.

The second approach, fidgeometric, measures the degree to
which the subject jars or vibrates the cage or platform on which
he is placed. For example, the ballistograph is an apparatus consisting of a cable or chain connected hydraulically to a recording
device sensitive to the subject's overt actions while in the chair.
Another frequently used instrument is the stabilimeter, an apparatus fashioned after the ballistograph. Sprague (1969) measured head movements by means of a stabilimeter, and telemetry to
classify children into higher and lower activity groups. Telemetry
is the use of instruments that remotely record behavior without
there being any physical and/or visual contact between the subject
and the experimenter. Sykes et al. (1971) used a stabilimetric
cushion designed like that of Sprague and Thorpe (1966) to compare motor restlessness between normal and hyperactive children.
Herron and Ransden (1967) also used radio telemetry for the
measurement of behavior from an appreciable distance and listed
the following advantages of such a technique: no encumbering
wire hookup, increased freedom of movement for the subject, the
presence of an observer is not required, and data can be collected
without the subject's awareness and cooperation. There appears
to be available a series of different techniques which for the most
part have been employed independently of a theoretical rationale.
This is not the case for all studies, but there is a large proportion
for which there is a lack of mutual interdependency between
methodology and behavior.

The interaction between the two dimensions of assessment
procedure and theoretical definition of the construct has been
represented as a matrix (Fig. 1). By examining the general framework of the matrix and taking into account research and comments presented earlier, some degree of closure might be obtain-
able as to the advantages and disadvantages of any one chosen cell.

This model does not assume a substantial number of studies within each cell. For example, while observational techniques apply effectively in assessing hyperactivity from any one of the four theoretical viewpoints, a mechanical device has yet to be proposed that measures underlying psychological processes. Such processes are inferred from overt behavior, but as pointed out earlier, some mechanical techniques are quite appropriate, such as the electroencephalograph, for assessing some organic dysfunction.

METHODOLOGICAL CONCERNS

Delong (1972) presents an interesting and valid position in reference to the measurement of hyperactivity. He writes that "it is axiomatic in psychological measurement that different means for measuring any specific behavior produce dissimilar results. Indeed the failure to standardize (and validate) measurement instruments has made it increasingly more difficult to understand hyperactivity and its etiology (p. 193). While Delong's warning may appear directed solely to those contemplating the use of paper and pencil assessment techniques, other observers have issued parallel concerns. Johnson (1971) in his study utilizing ultrasound and photoelectric cells comments that "observation of activity may differ from activity detected by various machines, causing disagreement in the conclusions reached by the different methodologies (p.2110)." He continued to warn investigators of hyperactivity of the "idiosyncracies" of the specific device being used, and that studies of activity level must take into account the limitations of the apparatus employed.

The paramount concern in any discussion of measurement is the question of validity. Our presentation and consideration of hyperactivity clearly points to two general issues. First, there exists a broad variety of assumed causal definitions of hyperactivity, and second, regardless of one's definition, there appears to be a limitless number of methods to measure this behavior. This pattern of broad definitional variability has been illustrated in the matrix presented earlier. We believe that a direct means of resolving the issue of validity as it relates to the construct of hyperactivity is found in the writing of Campbell and Fiske (1959). These authors have provided a model for validity identified as a multitrait-multi-method paradigm. They discuss how any assessment device is really a trait-method unit. That is, a particular test (device) measures a given trait using a single method. In order to fully understand the relative contributions of the trait and the method components to the assessment score, more than one trait and more than one method must be studied. What is actually being investigated then is the convergent and discriminant validity of the trait, where convergent validity is shown by the high correlation between same traits measured by different methods and discriminant validity is established by showing that the different traits are not highly interrelated, even when assessed using the same procedure. A discussion of convergent and discriminant validity is then established by showing that the different traits are not highly interrelated, even when assessed using the same procedure. A discussion of convergent and discriminant validity taking into consideration the two dimensions earlier discussed provides a perspective from which to evaluate the assessment procedure incorporated. Through such an examination of the validity of the procedure the foundation is presented for a more valid consistent evaluation of what is termed *hyperactivity.*

In addition, regardless of the theoretical definition of the syndrome, the researcher should strive to use an instrument that ideally is (1) nonobstrusive in that the use of the instrument itself does not alter the nature of the phenomenon being studied, (2) inconspicuous in that the subject being measured is not aware of the assessment taking place (often a limiting factor in the mechanical means of measurement), and (3) relatively inexpensive and portable. It should of course maintain a high degree of reliability across situations for which it was designed and be valid within the context for which it was intended.

CONCLUSION

This chapter is an attempt to discuss some of the current trends and issues in the measurement of hyperactivity as well as to suggest future directions in the development of measurement instruments. Although such a menage of terms and different perspectives might at first seem difficult and somewhat removed from everyday concerns, it is upon such building blocks the authors feel valid and reliable measures of hyperactivity can be developed. The classroom teacher, however, is seldom in the position to act as a researcher either on a full or part-time basis, and consequently is dependent upon research and findings as reported by others to do what is best for the child. Being aware of what is contained in the literature and the issues which are involved in the measurement of hyperactivity will provide interested individuals with the necessary foundation to better understand the term *hyperactivity* and to later apply skills and techniques appropriate for this special type of child. Too often intuitions are trusted rather than available information with the result being well-intentioned, but misguided actions. Due to the ambiguous nature of the meaning and measurement of hyperactivity, from its diagnosis to its treatment, all those concerned and/or working with such children must make a serious attempt to expose themselves to all the available information on the hyperactive child. The child's behavior then becomes appreciably more understandable and allows for the use of tried and tested principles and practices to maximize services and meet the child's needs.

REFERENCES

Aronson, L. J.: The psychologist and minimal brain dysfunction: Ten steps to maximum incompetence. *Ment Hyg, 55:*523-525, 1971.

Battle, E., and Lacey, B.: A context for hyperactivity in children over time. *Child Devel, 43:*757-773, 1972.

Bell, R. O.: Adoption of small wrist watches for mechanical recording of activity in infants and children. *J Exp Child Psychol, 6:*302-305, 1968.

Bell, R. Q., Waldrop, M. F., and Weller, G.M.: A rating system for the assessment of hyperactive and withdrawn children in preschool samples. *Am J Orthopsychiatry, 42:*23-24, January, 1972.

Buddenhagen, R. G., and Sickler, P.: Hyperactivity: A forty-eight hour sample plus a note on etiology. *Am J Ment Defic, 73:*580, 1969.

Campbell, D.: Motor activity in a group of newborn babies. *Biol Neonate, 13:*257-270, 1968.

Campbell, D. T., and Fiske, D. W.: Convergent and discriminant validation by the multitrait-multimethod matrix. *Psychol Bull, 56:*81-105, 1959.

Cantwell, D. P.: Psychiatric illness in the families of hyperactive children. *Arch Gen Psychiatry, 27,* 1972.

Chalfant, J. C., and Scheffelen, M. A.: Cerebral Processing Dysfunctions in Children: A Review of the Research. HEW, NONDS Monograph No. 9, 1969.

Chess, S.: Diagnosis and treatment of the hyperactive child. *NY State J Med, 60:*2379-2385, 1959.

Clements, S. D.: Minimal brain dysfunction in children. HEW, NINDB, Monograph No. 3, 1966.

Clemmens, R. L., and Kenny, D.: Clinical correlates of learning disabilities. Minimal brain dysfunction and hyperactivity. *Clin Pediatr, 11:*311-313, 1972.

Connors, C. K.: A teacher rating scale for use in drug studies with children. *Am J Psychol, 126:*884-888, 1969.

Conrad, W. G., and Dusell, J.: Anticipating the response to amphetamine therapy in the treatment of hyperactive children. *Pediatrics, 40:*96-98, 1967.

Cromwell, R. L., Baumeister, A., and Hawkins, W. F.: Research in activity level. In Ellis, N. R. (Ed.): *Handbook of Mental Deficiency.* New York, McGraw, 1963, 632-663.

Cromwell, R. L., Dalk, B. E., and Foshee, J. G.: The relationships among eyelid conditioning, intelligence, activity level and age. *Am J Ment Defic, 65:*744-748, 1961.

DeLong, Arthur: What have we learned from psychoactive drug research on hyperactives? *Am J Dis Child, 123,* 1972.

Demetroff, M. L.: Motor skills of hyperactive children. *Am J Orthopsychiatry, 42:*746, 1972.

Dildine, G. C.: Energy-Basis of living and learning. *Natl Ed Assoc J XXXIX:* 252-253, 1950.

Douglas, V. I.: Stop, look and listen: The problem of sustained attention and impulse control in hyperactive and normal children. *Can J Beh Sci, 4:*(4), 1972.

Foshee, J. G.: Studies in activity level: 1. Simple and complex task performance in defectives. *Am J Ment Defic, 62:*882-886, 1958.

Grunewald-Zuberbier, E.: Telemetric measurement of motor activity in maladjusted children under different experimental conditions. *Psychiat Neurol Neurochil, 75:*371-B, September-October, 1972 (Netherlands Society of Psychiatry and Neurology).

Halverson, C. F., and Waldrop, M. F.: The relations of mechanically recorded activity level to varieties of preschool behavior. *Child Devel, 44:* 678-681, 1973.

Herron, R. E., and Ramsden, R. W.: Continuous monitoring of overt human body movement by radio telemetry: A brief review. *Percept Mot Skills, 24:*1303-1308, 1967.

Herron, R. E., and Ramsden, R. W.: A telepedometer for remote measurement of human locomotor activity. *Psychophysiology, 4*:112-115, 1967.

Howell, M. C.: Hyperactivity in children: Types, diagnosis, drug therapy, approaches to management. *Clin Pediatr, 11*:30-39, 1972.

Hutt, C.: A method for the study of children's behavior. *Devel Med Child Neurol, 5*:233-245, 1963.

Ingram, T. T. S.: A characteristic form of onerative behavior in brain damaged children. *J Ment Sci, 102*:550, 1956.

Johnson, C. F.: Limits on measurement of activity level in children using ultrasound and photoelectric cells. *Am J Ment Defic, 77*:301-310, 1972.

Johnson, C. F.: Activity Measurement in Children — A Review. Unpublished manuscript, 1972b.

Johnson, C. F.: Hyperactivity and the machine: The actometer. *Child Devel, 42*:2105-2110, 1971.

Kaspar, J. C., and Lowenstein, R.: The effect of social interaction on activity levels in 6-8 year old boys. *Child Devel, 42*:1294-1298, 1971.

Kenny, T. J., Clemmens, R. L., Hudson, B. W., Lentz, G. A., Cicci, R., and Nair, P.: Characteristics of children referred because of hyperactivity. *J Pediatr, 79*:618-622, 1971.

Keogh, B.: Hyperactivity and learning disorders: Review and speculation. *Except Child,* 101-109, October, 1971.

Laufer, M. W., Denhoff, E., and Solomons, G.: Hyperkinetic behavior syndrome in children. *J Pediatr, 50*:463-474, 1957.

Lesser, L. L.: Hyperkinesis in children. Operational approach to management. *Clin Pediatr, 9*:548-552, September, 1970.

Loo, C., and Wenar, C.: Activity level and motor inhibition: Their relationship to intelligence test performance in normal children. *Child Devel, 42*:967-971, 1971.

Maccoby, E. E., Dowley, E. M., Hagen, J. W., and Degerman, R.: Activity level and intellectual functioning in normal and preschool children. *Child Devel, 36*:761-770, 1965.

McConnell, T. C., and Cromwell, R. L.: Studies in activity level: VII effects of amphetamine drug administration on the activity level of retarded children. *Am J Ment Defic, 68,* March, 1964.

Minde, K., Webb, G., and Sykes, D.: Studies on the hyperactive child: Parental and paranatal factors associated with hyperactivity. *Devel Med Child Neurol, 10*:355-363, 1968.

Morgan, C. T., and Stellar, E.: *Physiological Psychology.* New York, McGraw, 1950.

Morrison, J. R., and Stewart, M. A.: A family study of the hyperactive child syndrome. *Biol Psychiatry, 3*:189-195, 1971.

Palkes, J., and Stewart, M.: Intellectual ability and performance of hyperactive children. *Am J Orthopsychiatry, 42*:35-39, 1972.

Pope, L., and Pope, M.: Measurement of motor activity in human subjects. *Percept Mot Skills, 29*:315-319, 1969.

Pope, L.: Motor activity in brain injured children. *Am J Orthopsychiatry, 40*(5):783-794, 1970.

Reed, J. D.: Spontaneous activity of animals: A review of the literature since 1929. *Psychol Bull, 44*:393-412, 1947.

Routh, D. K., and Roberts, R. D.: Minimal brain dysfunction in children: failure to find evidence for a behavioral syndrome. *Psychol Rep, 31*:307-314, 1972.

Schmitt, B., Martin, H. P., Nellhaus, G., Cravens, J., Camp, B. W., and Jordan, K.: The hyperactive child. *Clin Pediatr, 12*:154-169, 1973.

Schmitt, B. D.: The Hyperactive Child. Paper read at the University of Kansas Medical Center, June, 1974.

Schulman, J. L., Kaspar, J. C., and Throne, F. M.: *Brain Damage and Behavior*. Springfield, Thomas, 1965.

Schulman, J. L., and Reisman, J. M.: An objective measure of hyperactivity. *Am J Ment Defic, 64*:455-456, 1959.

Sprague, R. L.: Psychotropic Drug Effects on Learning and Activity Level of Children. Unpublished manuscript, 1969.

Sprague, R. L., and Toppe, L. K.: Relationship between activity level and delay of reinforcement in the retarded. *J Exp Child Psychol, 3*:390-397, 1966.

Stewart, M., Pitts, F. N., Craig, A. G., and Dieruf, W.: The hyperactive child syndrome. *Am J Orthopsychiatry, 36*:861-867, 1966.

Sykes, D. H., Douglas, V. I., Weiss, G., and Minde, K.: Attention in hyperactive children and the effect of methylphenedate (Ritalin). *J Child Psychol Psychiatry, 12*:129-139, 1971.

Victor, J. B., Halverson, C. F., and Buczkowski, H. J.: Objective behavior measures of first and second grade boys free play and teacher ratings in a behavior problem checklist. *Psychol Schools, 4*:439-443, 1973.

Werry, J. S.: Diagnosis, etiology, and treatment of hyperactivity in children. *Learning Disorders, 3*, Special Child Publication, Washington, D. C., 1968.

Willerman, L., and Plomen, R.: Activity level in children and their parents. *Child Devel, 44*:854-858, 1973.

Wright, H.: Observational child study. In Mussen, P. H. (Ed.): *Handbook of Research Methods in Child Development*. New York, Wiley, 1960.

Zruli, J. R., Westman, J. C., Arthur, B., and Rice, B.: Our evaluation of methodology used in the study of psychoactive drugs for children. *Am Acad Child Psychiatry, 5*:284-291, 1966.

Annotated bibliography

Richard L. Simpson

THE HYPERACTIVE CHILD: RESOURCES

HYPERACTIVITY IN CHILDREN, known and described in medical and behavioral literature since the early 1920's, is a conspicuous complaint made by adults about children's behavior, particularly in educational settings. Estimates as high as 10 percent of school age children between the ages of six and twelve are included in this category of psychopathology. Although definitions vary, hyperactivity is agreed to include bodily movements which place the child's level of activity at the upper end of the distribution of this behavioral trait. Since reliable and valid measurements of activity have proven to be a difficult task, no exact definition of the hyperactive child in terms of a measured quantity of movement or activity has yet been made. Consequently, definitions of such children have been of an operational nature. The *Diagnostic and Statistical Manual* of the American Psychiatric Association categorizes this disorder, for example, as a syndrome characterized by overactivity, restlessness, distractibility, short attention span, excitability, lability of mood, cognition problems and sometimes specific types of learning difficulties.

Numerous terms have been formulated to describe this relatively common disorder in children, although none seem to be totally satisfactory. *Minimal brain damage, hyperactive child, hyperkinetic syndrome* and *minimal cerebral dysfunction* are only a few of the terms proposed to describe the phenomena. In spite of the large number of reports dealing with the problems of hyperactivity, few studies have drawn definitive conclusions. However, the basic inferences of these studies have been unequivocally that little evidence exists to support this phenomena as a single homogeneous syndrome.

Although etiology has been attributed to numerous factors, little evidence exists to support a single source. The earliest reports on hyperactivity viewed the phenomena as brain damage, specifically resulting from encephalitis, trauma or anoxia. Of significance is the fact that an assumption of some type of organic etiology, albeit obscure, has been made and that hyperactivity is the single most salient diagnostic sign. Research designed to analyze this etiological hypothesis has typically been of such quality as to provide little empirical support. Because the label *cerebral dysfunction* has come to embrace so heterogeneous an agglomeration of children, many professionals suggest that it may be a designation having little clinical or educational worth. Basically, empirical data seems to support the contention that hyperactivity can and does occur many times in the absence of any organic pathology.

Although longitudinal studies are lacking with this population, present data suggests that hyperactivity decreases as a function of age and will usually disappear by the time the child reaches puberty. Even in view of this long-term positive prognosis, the chronic and disruptive nature of the pathology usually warrants some type of therapeutic intervention, particularly in the primary and intermediate grades at school. The purpose of the present annotated bibliography is to review literature related to not only hyperactivity but also the various therapeutic intervention techniques that have been employed to deal with the hyperactive child in educational settings. The bibliography will be structured around general characteristics and issues, measuring hyperactivity, drug intervention techniques and the use of behavioral techniques with the hyperactive child.

General Characteristics and Issues

Anderson, W.W.: The hyperkinetic child: A neurological appraisal. *Neurology, 13:*968-973, 1963.

A report on thirty hyperkinetic children between the ages of eight and twelve who were administered neurological, psychological and EEG evaluations revealed neurological abnormalities in a majority of the children. In virtually every case there were problems manifested in visual perception and visual motor integration. It was theorized that the hyperkinetic syndrome is related to a lack of perceptual motor integration and to minimal brain dysfunction.

Ayres, A.J.: Tactile functions: Their relation to hyperactive and perceptual motor behavior. *Am J Occup Ther, 18:*6-11, 1964.

A hypothesis was presented for explaining the hyperkinetic syndrome. It was suggested that two afferent systems, one a protective system which responds to stimuli with movement and alertness, and second a discriminative system—a cognitive system which interprets the nature of stimuli, are in a state of imbalance in the hyperactive child. According to the position presented, the hyperkinetic child either loses or never attains a balance between the two systems, causing the protective system to predominate. This is used to explain the distractible behavior and poor perceptual motor functioning found in children who are diagnosed as hyperactive.

Bax, M.: The active and overactive school child. *Devel Med Child Neurol, 14:*83-36, 1972.

In another study the role of the physician in the treatment and diagnosis of the overactive and hyperkinetic child was presented. It was noted that the physician's main responsibilities are in the area of diagnosing those specific areas in which the child has his greatest degree of difficulty and, in general, providing leadership in aiding the overactive, hyperkinetic child to adapt. Under specific discussion were the factors associated with psychiatric disorders, specific learning disabilities, educational endeavors, social history, cultural history, educational milieu and strategies for meeting the needs of the hyperactive child.

Burks, H.F.: The hyperkinetic child. *Except Child, 27*:18-26, 1960.

A rating scale was employed to evaluate the general procedures that are used to diagnose the hyperkinetic syndrome and to analyze the possible relationship between brain pathology and the associated behavior problems of the hyperkinetic syndrome. A rating scale which was standardized on 524 school age children in grades kindergarten through eight was used to evaluate symptoms such as overactivity, impulsivity, short attention span, perceptual cognitive difficulties and social, emotional and behavioral patterns. Those children, identified as hyperkinetic, were compared with normal subjects on EEG patterns, neuropsychiatric evaluations, developmental histories, psychological testing, neurochemistry and neurological examinations. On the basis of positive signs on the part of the hyperkinetic sample in the areas of the EEG evaluation, neuropsychiatric evaluations, developmental histories, psychiatric evaluations and the positive effect of chemotherapy on the behavioral patterns of the children, it was inferred that the characteristics commonly associated with the hyperkinetic syndrome can be traced to organic brain impairment. Specific educational techniques were outlined to deal with hyperkinetic children having this etiological foundation.

Cantwell, D.P.: Psychiatric illness in the families of hyperactive children. *Arch Gen Psychiatry, 27*:414-417, 1972.

A systematic evaluation of the parents of hyperactive children revealed a significant prevalence of certain mental disorders. The parents of fifty hyperactive children who were interviewed tended to show a far greater prevalence of alcoholism, hysteria and sociopathic behaviors than the parents of matched controls. In addition, a number of parents of hyperactive children were found to be hyperactive themselves as children.

Clements, S., and Peters, J.: Minimal brain dysfunction in the school age child. *Arch Child Psychiatry, 6:*185-197, 1963.

The need for professionals to evaluate conditions of minimal brain dysfunction as an etiological explanation for behavioral and academic problems was stressed. It was noted that in many cases child guidance clinic personnel tend to overlook subtle organic deviations in their efforts to obtain signs of psychogenesis. Specifically, it was noted that the symptoms that professionals should be most cognizant of are specific learning deficits, perceptual motor deficits, general coordination deficits, hyperkinesis, impulsivity, emotional lability, short attention span and/or distractibility, equivocal neurological signs and borderline abnormal or abnormal EEG patterns. Strategies for treating the minimally brain-damaged child were also outlined.

Cruickshank, W.N., Bentzen, F.A., Ratzeburg, F.H., and Tannhauser, N.T.: *A Teaching Method for Brain Injury and Hyperactive Children.* Syracuse, Syracuse U Pr, 1971.

In addition to confirming that environmental stimuli can distract hyperactive children, specific teaching suggestions were offered. In general, environmental stimuli were suggested to be an important variable in educating hyperactive children. Specifically, physical features such as walls, woodwork, floors and furniture were noted to be possible stimuli that could evoke responses incompatible with teaching. Thus, it was suggested that the child's learning environment be as devoid of competing stimuli as possible. The specific teaching methods included reducing environmental stimuli, reducing the physical space that a child has to operate in (one component of this teaching method is to use cubicles to control the amount of stimulation), operating a structured educational program and life arrangement and increasing the stimulus value of teaching materials.

Eisenzenberg, L.: The management of the hyperkinetic child. *Devel Med Child Neurol, 8:*593-598, 1966.

Hyperactivity in childhood is referred to as motor activity in excess of the range normal for age and sex. Although no statistical evidence was provided, it was reported that parents of hyperactive children feel their children to be restless and irritable as infants and to begin running as soon as they can walk. This combination of boundless energy and poor judgment requires that the child be supervised by the parent constantly. Educators also report these children to be seemingly unable to sit still, to be constantly on the go, to be unable to focus on any one activity, and to be unable to conform to the requirements of class discipline. Rather than the quantitative degree of movement in hyperactive children, it is suggested that the problem lies in the random and goalless nature of the child's activity and in his inability to inhibit responses to external or internal cues. It was also suggested that successful managment of the child requires full pediatric, neurological, psychological and educational disciplines coordinating their efforts in a way most beneficial to the hyperactive child.

Hertzig, M.E., Bortner, M., and Birch, H.G.: Neurologic findings in children educationally designated as brain damaged. *Am J Orthopsychiatry, 39(3)*:437-446, 1969.

One hundred and five children with a history of academic failure and/or maladjustment as well as independent confirmation of a diagnosis of brain damage were evaluated. Findings indicated that "hard signs" were found no more frequently among hyperactive children than among those who did not exhibit such behavioral disturbance. Although the hyperactive children were found to have a significantly greater number of "soft signs," the types of signs were not different from those found in nonhyperactive children. It was concluded that the clinical-neurological findings in the hyperactive children were qualitatively indistinguishable from nonhyperactive children, although the sample did provide clinical evidence of central nervous system abnormalities. Even so, it was noted that the designation of cerebral dysfunction did not directly define symptomatology, treatment or prognosis, and was therefore felt to be inappropriate for defining neurologic, behavioral or educational strategies.

Kenny, T.J., Clemmens, R.L., Hudson, B.W., Lentz, G.A., Cicci, R., Nair, P.: Characteristics of children referred because of hyperactivity. *J Pediatr, 79*:618-622, 1971.

Data were presented on one hundred children referred to an interdisciplinary clinic because of hyperactivity problems. Each of the one hundred children received a complete multidisciplinary evaluation. In independent observations by the professional staff, only approximately 25 percent of the children were judged to be excessively active. Only 13 percent of the subjects were rated as hyperactive by all of the diagnostic observers, while another 58 percent were judged to be not hyperactive by all of the staff. Conclusions drawn from this interesting study were that the behavioral pattern of hyperactivity is a poorly defined and inconsistent phenomena which is extremely difficult to diagnose even under multidisciplinary evaluation conditions. Of interest was the suggestion by this medical team that the assessment and management of hyperactive children be directed around behavioral and psychoeducational factors rather than medical techniques and that educators assume a greater role in controlling and coordinating the research efforts for the hyperactive child.

Keogh, B.K.: Hyperactivity and learning problems: Implications for teachers. *Educ Dig, 37:*45-47, 1971.

A review of definitions and symptoms of hyperactivity for the classroom teacher was presented. In addition, three hypotheses regarding the learning problems manifested by most hyperactive children and the teaching strategies which may be appropriate with this group of students were also reviewed.

Keogh, B.K.: Hyperactivity in learning disorders: Review and speculation. *Except Child, 38:*101-109, 1971.

A review of research on the hyperactive child was presented with the aim of specifying a relationship between this behavioral pattern and learning disabilities. In addition, a theoretical explanation was offered for the learning problems that are many times manifested by hyperactive children. It was suggested that these theoretical educational explanations are in need of empirical evaluation.

Laufer, M.W., and Denhoff, E.: Hyperkinetic behavior syndrome in children. *J Pediatr, 50:*463-474, 1975.

Laufer and Denhoff specified the basic symptoms of the hyperkinetic syndrome—hyperactivity, short attention span, poor concentration, variability in performance, impulsiveness, inability to delay impulse gratification, irritability and poor academic performance. They also specified that frequently hyperactive children manifest problems in infancy, school problems, sleep disturbances and, in some cases, mild emotional disturbances. Among those intervention procedures identified were drug intervention techniques, especially central nervous system stimulant drugs, special education and psychotherapy. This article specifically emphasized the need for psychological guidance for parents of hyperactive children and the need in some cases for psychotherapy for the children themselves.

Lucus, A., Rodin, E., and Simon, C.: Neurological assessment of children with early school problems. *Devel Med Child Neurol,* 7:145-146, 1965.

In an effort to investigate the developmental-neurological norms of various age groups and the meaning of deviations in motor performance and perceptual functioning, seventy-two antisocial, withdrawn and hyperactive children who had been referred for special educational placement were investigated. Data on the subjects was taken in the areas of personal and family history, psychiatric history, neurological, EEG, psychological and educational areas. Results indicated that the antisocial and withdrawal patterns of behavior and little or no relationship to neurological, EEG, intellectual or perceptual abnormalities. It was reported, however, that the symptom of hyperactivity, when present to the extent that it interfered grossly with school functioning, did appear to be related to findings of poor general motor coordination, motor difficulties and abnormal movements on the neurological exam. It was concluded that a neurological dysfunction can be correlated with hyperactivity, or it can be a manifestation of a developmental or integrational deficit.

Morrison, J.R., and Stewart, M.: A family study of the hyperactive child syndrome. *Biol Psychiatry, 3:*189-195, 1971.

In an investigation of the hypothesis that the hyperactive syndrome is a genetic trait, fifty children who had been diagnosed as hyperactive were compared with a matched nonhyperactive group. Data were solicited from each of the parents of the subjects in the areas of alcoholic usage in the family, psychotic and character disorder patterns in the family, and whether or not the parents themselves had been hyperactive as children Results indicated that the hyperactive syndrome appears to be passed from one generation to another with a great deal of consistency. In addition, it appears that the condition of hyperactivity is closely correlated with specific disorders in the parents. Conclusions regarding whether this was a modeling or genetic outcome were not drawn.

Palkes, J., Stewart, M., and Kahana, B.: Porteus maze performance of hyperactive boys after training in self-directed verbal commands. *Child Devel, 39*:817-826, 1968.

Twenty hyperactive school-aged males of normal intelligence were reported to gain voluntary selfcontrol over their hyperactive behavior through a program of self-directed verbal commands. Porteus maze performance was employed as the major dependent measure, and this particular instrument was used both as a pre and posttest. The data suggest that training in self-directed verbal commands may be an effective technique for modifying the hyperactive behavior of school age children.

Renshaw, D.C.: *The Hyperactive Child.* Chicago, Nelson-Hall, 1974.

. In a blending of experimental, clinical and educational information, the characteristics of the hyperactive child and intervention approaches for dealing with this disability were reviewed. The basic assumption underlying this discussion was that the etiology of hyperactivity is based on a specific neurological malfunction.

Rodin, E., Lucus, A., and Simon, C.: A study of behavior disorders in children by means of general purpose computers. *Proceeding of the Conference on Data Acquisition and Processing in Biological Medicine.* Oxford, Pergamon, 1963.

Rodin et al.'s study reported a factor analytic analysis on the association between historical neurological, electronencephalographic, perceptual-cognitive and behavioral measures in a group of seventy-two school age children referred by school authorities because of behavior and/or academic problems. The results of the study indicated several apparently independent clinical dimensions. The first of these dimensions was motor incoordination, consisting mainly of impaired sensory motor coordination. Other clinical signs related to the intelligence of the seventy-two subjects, maturational variables, abnormal EEG patterns, hyperactivity and antisocial behavior. Conclusions drawn from this study were that the syndrome of minimal brain damage is a single cause, mainly organistic. It was also noted that since the study lacked a normal control group it was somewhat difficult to ascertain whether the observed findings are typical for children diagnosed as minimally brain damaged or whether it reflects a general developmental pattern.

Schmitt, B.D., Martin, H.P., Nellhaus, G., Cravens, J., Camp, B.W., and Jordan, K.: The hyperactive child. *Clin Pediatr,* *12*(3):154-169, 1973.

A medical and psychological discussion of the subtypes of hyperactive child, the etiology of hyperactivity and the use of various intervention techniques was presented by Schmitt et al. The article pointed out that there was an acute lack of data supporting the presence of brain damage as a salient variable in explaining hyperactivity. It was suggested that professionals need to examine more productive areas in, evaluating the causes of hyperactivity. In the area of drug intervention techniques it was emphasized that medication can only be employed as an adjunct to other aspects of therapy.

Schrager, J., Lindy, J., Harrison, S., McDermott, J., and Killins, E.: The hyperkinetic child: Some consensually validated behavioral correlates. *Except Child, 32*(9):635-637, 1966.

In a multidisciplinary survey on the hyperkinetic child, a fifty-five-item behavioral checklist was completed by teachers, psychologists, psychiatrists, social workers and pediatricians. The results indicated good interdisciplinary agreement concerning the behavioral charcteristics of the hyperkinetic syndrome. Seventy-five percent of the individuals completing the behavioral checklist indicated that the behaviors primarily seen in the hyperkinetic syndrome are restlessness, inattention, an inability to sit still, easy distractibility and a low frustration tolerance. It was concluded that even though there are differences in the etiology and meaning of the symptoms in the hyperkinetic syndrome, there is a high degree of agreement within disciplines as to the nature of the signs and symptoms.

Sprague, R.L., and Toppe, L.K.: Relationship between activity level and a way of reinforcement in the retarded. *J Exp Child Psychol, 3*:390-397, 1966.

Hyperactive retarded children were found to be significantly poorer on a two-choice discrimination task than matched nonhyperactive retardates. Specifically, the low active retardate group was able to give significantly more correct responses in the learning trials than was the high active group. It was concluded that the greater amount of movement shown by the hyperactive sample may cause them to move away from the stimulus and reinforcement, thus lowering performance.

Stewart, M.A., and Olds, S.W.: *Raising a Hyperactive Child.* New York, HarRow, 1973.

Stewart and Olds' book was written for parents, attention being directed toward specifying the nature of the problems caused by hyperactive children and offering specific advice for handling children of this type. A significant aspect of this book is the ability that it seems to have in reducing the negative affect of parents of exceptional children by suggesting that their responsibility for the problem may be minimal. It presents a logical case for replacing these negative feelings with specific techniques for reducing hyperactivity.

Stewart, N.A., Pitts, F.N., Craig, A.G., and Dieruf, W.: The hyperactive child syndrome. *Am J Orthopsychiatry, 36*:861-867, 1966.

In an attempt to obtain systematic data on the symptoms and histories of hyperactive children, the life histories of thirty-seven hyperactive subjects were compared with those of thirty-six normal subjects. Data on the schoolage, preadolescent population was obtained by interviewing the mothers of the subjects. Among the findings was a lack of evidence for a specific etiological factor for the hyperactivity. In addition, evidence of the influence of prenatal or perinatal vari-

ables, and evidence of extreme variability in school work and behavior was reported. It was also reported by many of the mothers that
the hyperactivity symptoms began in infancy. On the basis of this report it was concluded that those mothers who indicated that their children did not display symptoms of hyperactivity until beginning school
either represented extremely chaotic homes or tended to blame the
school for all of the child's difficulties.

Strauss, A.A., and Lehtinen, L.E.: *Brain Injured Child.* New York,
Grune, 1947.

A landmark study by Strauss and Lehtinen defined the brain injured child as having characteristics similar to those characterizing the
hyperactive child. It was suggested that the brain injured child is ab-
normally responsive to stimuli in the environment. When such a child
is placed in situations of constant stimulation, he meets the situation
with nonfunctional responses. To deal with this disability it was suggested that a child's learning materials be stripped to the barest essen-
tials. It is suggested that this allows the child to work with as few
distractions as possible.

Tizard, B.: Observations of over-active imbecile children in controlled and uncontrolled environments. I: Classroom studies.
*Am J Ment Defic, 32:*540-546, 1968.

In a study of two groups of matched severely retarded children,
one overactive and one not, it was noted that although the hyperactive subjects had a higher activity count, they had few other features
of the hyperkinetic syndrome. Specifically, the hyperactive retardates
did not differ from the nonhyperactive retardates on the dimension
of aggressiveness nor in the areas of developmental history, neurological signs of social deficits.

Waldrop, M.F., and Georing, J.D.: Hyperactivity and minor physical anomalies in elementary-school children. *Am J Orthopsychiatry, 41:*602-607, 1971.

In a project designed to correlate hyperactivity with physical
anomalies, it was predicted that children identified by educators as

hyperactive would have more physical anomalies than those children judged by educators as being nonhyperactive. This research hypothesis was tested using 775 pupils diagnosed as hyperactive. The research indicated that male hyperactives had more physical anomalies than their nonhyperactive counterparts, but their relationship was not true for girls. It was suggested by these researchers that since hyperactivity may be linked to certain congenital variables, educators and other professionals should be more sympathetic and appreciative of the difficulties that hyperactive children have in controlling their behavior. It was also suggested that this relationship of increased physical anomalies at least in males, may serve as a predictor of hyperactive behavior in the future.

Weiss, G., Minde, K., Werry, J.S., Douglas, B., and Nemeth, E.: Studies on the hyperactive child: Five year follow-up. *Arch Gen Psychiatry, 24:*409-414, 1971.

Sixty-four severely handicapped, hyperactive children, most of whom had been diagnosed as minimally brain damaged, were evaluated in a longitudinal study. These adolescents were initially seen as children and were later evaluated as adolescents on behavioral, academic and neurological variables. Although it was reported that hyperactivity decreases with age, it was noted that the conditions of inattention, lack of concentration and poor school achievement remained. In addition, it was reported that even though the adolescents outgrow the overt quantitative hyperactivity pattern, they do continue to encounter interpersonal and psychiatric problems. Specifically, these problems consisted of emotional immaturity, an inability to maintain goals, poor self-images and social maladjustment.

Wender, P.H.: *The Hyperactive Child.* New York, Crown, 1973.

Wender's handbook, written expressly for parents of hyperactive children, reviews in specific but yet understandable language the characteristics, causes and treatment of hyperactivity. Special emphasis is given to the various therapeutic procedures that parents frequently ask questions about. Specifically, parents are offered aid in understanding the medical, psychological and educational procedures that are employed with the hyperactive child and his family.

Werry, J.S.: Studies on the hyperactive child. *Arch Gen Psychiatry*, *19*:9-16, 1968.

Employing a factor analysis approach, neurological, EEG, medical, historical, cognitive and psychiatric measures were evaluated in 103 hyperactive children. The factor analysis revealed ten unrelated dysfunctions in the sample employed. Inferences drawn from this study indicated that even multidisciplinary measures cannot tap a single dimension of minimal brain damage; rather, it appears that a series of developmental dimensions or a combination of dimensions may be impaired in the condition, minimal brain dysfunction. It was suggested that the conclusions regarding these functions and the interrelated nature of the variables cannot be easily analyzed.

Werry, J.S., Minde, K., Guzman, A., Weiss, G., Dogan, K., and Hoy, E.: Studies on the hyperactive child VII: Neurological status compared with neurotic and normal children. *Am J Orthopsychiatry, 42*(3):441-450, 1972.

Twenty hyperactive children between the ages of six and twelve were compared on neurological variables with a matched sample of nonhyperactive neurotic and normal children. Although there were no significant differences on the medical histories, EEG records or major neurological areas, the hyperactive children were found to possess significantly more *soft neurological signs* than the other groups. It was suggested that hyperactivity in most children is a discreet form of psychopathology and that it may in many cases be an aspect of an organic syndrome.

Werry, J.S., and Sprague, R.L.: Hyperactivity. In Costello, C.G. (Ed.) : *Symptoms of Psychopathology*. New York, Wiley, 1970.

A concise overview of the etiology, assessment and remediation of hyperactivity was given. Of special interest is the attention which is given the evaluation and assessment of hyperactivity and the applicability of these techniques to educational settings.

Werry, J.S., Weiss, G., and Douglas, B.: Studies on the hyperactive child: Some preliminary findings. *Can Psychiatric Assoc, 9*:120-130, 1964.

A comparison of twenty-eight hyperactive subjects between the ages of seven and twelve with a matched sample of nonhyperactive children was conducted to determine if minimal brain damage is a significant variable in accounting for hyperactivity. Results indicated that there appears to be a tendency for more hyperactive than normal children to have a history of accidents in the pregnancy, delivery and postnatal period, which could possibly be linked with brain damage. Conclusions drawn from this study were that chronic hyperactivity is not exclusively caused by brain damage, although this may be one of the possible contributing agents. Other etiological variables isolated were the innate activity level of a given child, the anxiety level of given hyperactive children and aberrant maturational development.

The Measurement of Hyperactivity

Bass, N.H., and Schulman, J.L.: Quantitative assessment of children's activity in and out of bed. *Am J Dis Child, 113:*242-244, 1967.

A comparison of activity levels in two groups of hospitalized boys by means of an actometer attached to the wrists and ankles of the subjects was described by Bass and Schulman (1967). The comparison between the bedrest children and the subjects who were up and about revealed no statistically significant differences, indicating that allowing children activity on certain days made no significant differences in their later activity levels. Implications for early ambulation of hospitalized children were discussed.

Bell, R.Q.: Adaption of small wristwatches for mechanical recording of activity in infants and children. *J Exp Child Psychol, 6:* 302-305, 1968.

A method for differentiating various activity components through the use of small modified actometers designed to tap movements across the axis of the body was reported. Normative data and test-retest reliability was given.

Bindra, D., and Blond, J.: A time-sample method for measuring general activity and its components. *Can J Psychol, 12:*74-76, 1958.

An adapted time-sample procedure was suggested as a means for obtaining activity measures on laboratory rats. The major modification in the described procedure was the use of descriptive rather than interpretative response categories. Pilot data were presented along with the note that this method can be most effectively utilized in combination with a stabilimeter and activity wheel apparatus.

Brown, C.C., and Whitman, J.R.: Apparatus for measuring restricted ranges of linear movement. *Am J Psychol, 76*:138-139, 1963.

A device for measuring linear movement through converting motion to electrical output which was capable of being picked up by a fixed transmitter was presented by Brown and Whitman. The movement, electrically picked up, was permanently recorded. It was noted that this device had the advantage of not interfering with the subjects' free movements.

Campbell, B.A.: Design and reliability of a new activity recording device. *J Comp Physiol Psychol, 47*:90-92, 1954.

A description of a device consisting of a balanced wire mesh cage that was designed to record spontaneous activity in rats was provided by Campbell (1954). Reliability and suggested uses for the device were also given.

Crawford, M.I., and Nicora, B.D.: Measurement of human group activity. *Psychol Rep, 15*:227-231, 1964.

An apparatus designed to measure human activity and a description of its use was presented. Thirty men, women and children were confined for eighty-six continuous hours in a community fall-out shelter under survival conditions. The relative activity for each subject was recorded hourly. Correlations between the ultrasonic activity measurement device and the observations of observers were high, suggesting that the apparatus may be a reliable method for acquiring data on human activity.

Ellis, N.R., and Pryer, R.S.: Quantification of gross bodily activity in children with severe oneuropathology. *Am J Ment Defic,* *63:*1034-1037, 1959.

A device designed to measure gross bodily movement in children was given. The apparatus consisted of an eight by eight-foot activity room which utilized a photronic principle to quantify movement. The room was crisscrossed with beams of light at two-foot intervals that were focused on a photoelectric cell mechanism on the other side of the room. A child's movement was able to break the light beam and the movement impulses were registered on a counter. The reliability of the apparatus as well as practical applications for the device were given.

Haworth, N.R., and Menolasciano, F.J.: Video taped observations of disturbed young children. *J Clin Psychol, 23:*135-140, 1967.

Haworth and Menolasciano reported on the development and use of a play interview designed to aid in the differential diagnosis of nonverbal children. The use of video-taping procedures during the play segments aided the clinicians in making appropriate types of analyses and eliminating the need for the clinicians to draw on-the-spot conclusions regarding their observations. These results and inferences were initially based on a sample of thirty-four children of various diagnoses (including normal) who were evaluated in the play interview. Inter and intrareliability score indicated the observational procedures under videotaped conditions to be quite reliable.

Herron, R.E., and Ramsden, R.W.: Continuous monitoring of overt human body movement by radio telemetry: A brief review. *Percept Mot Skills, 24:*1303-1308, 1967.

A method for measuring hyperactivity through radio transmitters placed on children such that bodily movements could be detected was reported. It was noted that the major difficulty in employing this particular measurement technique was designing suitable transducers to detect those dependent measures that the practitioners or researchers were most interested in.

Kessen, W., Hendry, L.S., and Leutzendorff, A.M.: Measurement of movement in the human newborn: A new technique. *Child Devel, 32:*95-105, 1961.

A novel technology for observing and analyzing the movements of infants using a motion picture procedure was described. It was noted that the procedure allowed for analysis of laterality variations, a deficiency in previous procedures of this type. A number of possible applications of the procedure were suggested.

Kibbler, G.O., and Richter, D.: Alpha rhythm and motor activity. *Electroencephalog Clin Neurophysiol, 2:*227, 1950.

Kibbler and Richter affirmed the assumption that voluntary muscle movements do in fact play a significant role in determining the phase of the alpha rhythm. It was suggested that even though the phase readings were not randomly distributed over all possible valves, they were variant for different subjects and the same subjects at different times.

Lee, D., and Hutt, C.: A playroom designed for filming children: A note. *J Child Psychol Psychiatry, 5:*263-265, 1964.

A description of a playroom designed to allow photography and the measurement of hyperactive children was provided. It was concluded that this is an economical and convenient way to obtain permanent records on children without distracting or modifying their typical hyperactive patterns.

Levitt, R.: An activity measure of sleeping and waking behavior. *Psychonomic Sci, 5:*287-288, 1966.

A small movement-detecting device capable of discriminating between sleeping and waking states in small animals was described. Activity, measured with an ultrasonic device, and sleep/waking states, measured by means of an EEG, revealed high correlation coefficients. It was concluded that the ultrasonic activity system can reliably be employed to detect sleep in small mammals.

Lipsitt, L.P., and DeLucia, C.A.: An apparatus for the measurement of specific response and general activity of the human neonate. *Am J Psychol, 73:*630-632, 1960.

An apparatus for measuring leg withdrawal behavior and general activity in the human neonate was described. The apparatus, a bed mounted on a spring balance and fulcrum in such a way that photo cells and light sources were activated with movement, permanently recorded all activity. Limitations and applications for employing these principles to measure other specific movements of bodily parts were also given.

Newberry, E.N.: Automatic measurement of general activity in time units. *Am J Psychol, 69:*655-659, 1956.

An apparatus which was able to divide equal time intervals and indicate on a permanent record whether activity had occurred during that time interval was offered. Although this apparatus was suggested for animal experimentation, it was noted that it has applications for other measurement problems.

Peacock, L.J., and Williams, N.: An ultrasonic device for recording activity. *Am J Psychol, 75:*648-652, 1962.

An electronic device was described which was ostensibly constructed to measure movement in an environment as large as a classroom. Since the apparatus contained no mechanical couplings between the subject and the system, the activity itself was not influenced by the device. A number of possible applications were suggested for the equipment described.

Sainsbury, P.: A method of measuring spontaneous movements by time sampling motion pictures. *J Ment Sci, 100:*742-748, 1954.

A method was described for measuring spontaneous movement through a time-sampling film procedure. It was suggested that this is a far more adequate observational procedure than direct observational techniques. Although the numbers that were employed in the investigation were small, the results indicated that this method can be a reliable and valid procedure.

Schulman, J.L., and Reisman, J.M.: An objective measure of hyperactivity. *Am J Ment Defic, 64:*455-456, 1959.

An apparatus for objectively measuring hyperactivity was described. This device, consisting of an automatically-winding wrist actometer was reported to have relatively high interwatch reliability. Specific applications for using the device with hyperactive children were suggested.

Drug Intervention with the Hyperactive Child

Arnold, L.E., Kirilcuk, W., Carson, S.A., and Carson, E.O.: Levo-amphetamine and dextroamphetamine: Differential effect on aggression and hyperkinesis in children and dogs. *Am J Psychiatry, 130:*165-170, 1973.

In an attempt to correlate the effects of various drugs with the differential diagnosis of hyperkinetic children, eleven differentially diagnosed children were evaluated. Results indicated that certain types of children are most amenable to specific types of drugs.

Bender, L., and Cottington, F.: The use of amphetamine sulfate (benzedrine) in child psychiatry. *Am J Psychiatry, 99:*116-121, 1942.

It was suggested that benzedrine can be a useful adjunct to the treatment of neurotic and hyperactive children because the medication can provide the child with a feeling of well-being. It was suggested that a child with this positive frame of mind is able to deal with his inner tensions and anxieties in a more socially appropriate manner.

Bradley, C.: The behavior of children receiving benzedrine. *Am J Psychiatry, 94:*577, 1973.

Bradley's was the first empirical report that amphetamines could be employed to alleviate behavioral disorders in children. Beneficial results in the area of school performance and behavior in residentially placed children of mixed etiology were reported. Not only did the central nervous system stimulant drug bring about improvement in school performance in approximately one-half the children, but the population of withdrawn, lethargic children tended to become more alert and displayed a pattern of happiness in social situations. This was the first report also of hyperactive and aggressive children becoming calmer while receiving the central nervous system stimulant medications.

Bradley, C., and Green, E.: Psychometric performance of children receiving amphetamine (benzedrine) sulfate. *Am J Psychiatry,* *97*:388-394, 1940.

Bradley and Green's was one of the first follow-up studies on the reported significant behavioral and academic changes that are within the scope of certain central nervous system stimulant drugs. This study reported that intelligence scores, as measured by the Stanford-Binet, were not significantly affected by the administration of amphetamine sulfate. It was inferred that the reported intellectual gains that are within the scope of benzedrine medication are a function of a child's improved emotional attitude towards his task.

Bradley, C., and Bowen, M.: School performance of children receiving amphetamine (benzedrine) sulfate. *Am J Orthopsychiatry,* *10*:782-788, 1940.

Significant academic improvement in nineteen institutionalized elementary school children was reported following the administration of amphetamine sulfate. The most significant improvement was in the area of mathematical performance. The effects on spelling performance were variable, with notable improvement in some cases and diminution of work in others.

Bradley, C., and Bowen, M.: Amphetamine (benzedrine) therapy of children's behavior disorders. *Am J Orthopsychiatry,* *11*:92-103, 1941.

A follow-up study by Bradley and Bowen (1941) on the effects of amphetamine sulfate was conducted with one hundred hospitalized problem children. This uncontrolled report indicated that 54 percent of the subjects became more subdued in their behavior; 21 percent failed to alter their activities; 19 percent increased their psychomotor stimulation; 6 percent showed improved scholastic performance without a behavior change; and 7 percent became clinically more of a problem.

Bradley, C.: Benzedrine and dexedrine in the treatment of children's behavior disorders. *Pediatrics, 5:*24-37, 1950.

Bradley, the original researcher with central nervous system stimulants, suggests that the effects of benzedrine and dexedrine are approximately equal. Uncontrolled data indicated that a large percentage of the children subjected to this treatment were more adequate in dealing with various situations. It was again affirmed that central nervous system stimulant drugs can be effective in altering a child's reaction to distressing situations.

Burks, H.F.: The hyperkinetic child. *Except Child, 27:*18-26, 1960.

Forty-three hyperactive/hyperkinetic children were rated on their behaviors by their classroom teachers before and after amphetamine therapy. The behavioral rating scales were designed to tape symptoms which were felt to be related to brain damage. Since the results indicated that the hyperactive children with abnormal EEG reading improved more than those with normal EEG readings it was suggested that the use of central nervous system stimulant drugs can be used most effectively with brain-damaged children.

Campbell, M.: Lithium and chlorpromazine: A controlled classroom study on hyperactive severely disturbed young children. *J Autism Child Schizo, 2:*234-263, 1972.

In a comparison study of the effects of chlorpromazine and lithium in hyperactive psychotic and nonpsychotic preschool children, subjects were evaluated under each of the two medications. The results yielded data indicating that there were no significant differences between the effects of lithium and chlorpromazine according to the ratings of a psychiatrist.

Campbell, S.B., Douglas, V.I., and Morgenstein, G.: Cognitive styles in hyperactive children and the effects of methylphenidate. *J Child Psychol Psychiatry, 12:*55-67, 1971.

Hyperactive children were reported to become more efficient problem solvers while under the effects of methylphenidate treatment. These hyperactive children were described as being more reflective and able to inhibit incorrect responses and to delay responding sufficiently to consider all possible responses while receiving the central nervous system stimulant drug. It was suggested that reports of improved school achievement and classroom behavior that are brought about by methylphenidate treatment may result from an increased ability to focus, organize and delay impulses.

Conners, C.K.: What parents need to know about stimulant drugs and special education. *J Learn Disabil, 6:*349-352, 1973.

Conners' 1973 study, which was ostensibly designed to evaluate the effectiveness of various forms of drug treatment, the physiological mechanism by which these medications act, and the positive academic and social effects that these medications can have, revealed several educational implications. First, it was noted that no particular diagnostic category of exceptional children seemed to profit most from drug therapy. In addition, it was emphasized that the effect of central nervous system stimulant medications is much more complex than had originally been thought. It was pointed out that these medications can no longer simply be perceived as a pharmacological means of reducing a child's activity level. Since not only the quantity, but the quality of the activity and the child's personality are also modified, the drugs obviously are quite complex in nature. It was also noted that the drug treament in and of itself cannot be the total therapeutic strategy but must be used in conjunction with other therapies. In addition, it was noted the special education teacher needs to maintain close contact with the physician who prescribed the drugs so that feedback can be provided on whether or not the medications helped to accomplish those goals which they were originally designed for.

Conners, C.K., and Eisenberg, L.: The effects of methylphenidate on symptomatology and learning in disturbed children. *Am J Psychiatry, 120:*458-464, 1963.

In a study of residentially placed children from two institutions, it was reported that subjects who received methylphenidate made significant progress, especially on overt behaviors that are frequently reported to be problems by aides. A forty-eight-item symptom checklist indicated significant differences between those subjects receiving the active medication and those receiving a placebo drug. It was also reported that significantly fewer errors were made on the Porteus-maze test under the influence of the methylphenidate.

Conners, C.K., Eisenberg, L., and Barcai, A.: Effect of dextroamphetamine on children. *Arch Gen Psychiatry, 17:*478-485, 1967.

In a double-blind crossover study conducted over a two-month period, fifty-two subjects with learning problems, many of whom were hyperactive, were evaluated under treatment conditions with dextroamphetamine sulfate and a placebo. In addition to improved teacher ratings, the subjects were reported to function significantly better on a battery of performance tests while on the active medication. These positive results were interpreted to be related to an increased degree of attentiveness and drive on the part of the children.

Conners, C.K., Eisenberg, L., and Sharpe, L.: Effects of methylphenidate (Ritalin) on paired-associate learning and Porteus-maze performance in emotionally disturbed children. *J Consult Psychol, 28:*14-22, 1964.

It was reported that methylphenidate offers suggestive, although not conclusive evidence, of being an aid to children in the area of paired associate performance and Porteus-Maze performance. In spite of the empirical results the investigators suggested that in view of the individual differences in responsiveness, the practical and/or clinical significance of central nervous system stimulant drugs must be further evaluated.

Conrad, W.G., Dworkin, E.S., Shai, A., and Tobiessen, J.E.: Effects of amphetamine therapy and prescriptive tutoring on the behavior and achievement of lower class hyperactive children. *J Learn Disabil, 9*(4):45-53, 1971.

In Conrad et al.'s evaluation of the long-term effect of dextroamphetamine on the behavior, achievement and perceptual cognitive functioning of hyperactive children, and the effects of drug and prescriptive perceptual-cognitive tutoring, it was reported that teacher and parent ratings were reflective of a reduction in hyperactivity and an improved ability to focus attention in children receiving the drug. Significantly greater improvement was reported in those hyperactive children who also received tutoring along with the medication. It was inferred from this finding that a tutorial experience can be employed in a positive manner along with drug therapy.

Conrad, W.G., and Insel, J.: Anticipating the response to amphetamine therapy in the treatment of hyperkinetic children. *Pediatrics, 40*:96-99, 1967.

It was suggested that children who respond most favorably to amphetamine therapy are those with a positive organic background, positive parent-child relationships and an absence of severe psychiatric problems. This uncontrolled study reported that 75 percent of the above-defined group improved significantly under the central nervous system stimulant therapy.

Delong, A.R.: What we have learned from psychoactive drug research on hyperactives. *Am J Dis Child, 123*:177-180, 1972.

Specific methodological considerations that need to be considered when doing drug research with hyperactive children are enumerated. These variables included a placebo control, blind procedures, random assignment of subjects to treatments, and of sufficient size to permit statistical analysis, a well-specified sample, precise measurement and criteria and an analysis of the social setting in which the children employed in the studies have been drawn. In addition, major questions which have been raised in the use of drug treatment were also dealt with. These included the issue of labeling the condition *hyperactivity,*

the etiology of the disorder, specific behaviors identified with hyperactivity, behavioral symptoms, classroom learning characteristics, related syndromes, measuring specific behaviors and the use of drug
medication.

Denhoff, E., Davids, A., and Hawkins, R.: Effects of dextroamphetamine on hyperkinetic children: A controlled double-blind
study. *J Learn Disabil, 9*(4):27-34, 1971.

A rating scale for evaluating hyperkinetic characteristics was reported to reveal favorable results from hyperactive and learning disabled children who were administered dextroamphetamine. Although
no significant differences in ratings were made in the area of improved
academic functioning, the teachers of the children did indicate that
the subjects were able to function more adequately under the active
drug conditions.

Eisenberg, L., Gilbert, A., Cytryn, L., and Molling, P.A.: The effectiveness of psychotherapy alone and in conjunction with
terphenazine or placebo in treatment of neurotic and hyperkinetic children. *Am J Psychiatry, 117*:1088-1093, 1971.

Hyperkinetic children were treated experimentally with a brief
period of psychotherapy, a brief period of psychotherapy plus a placebo treatment, or a brief period of psychotherapy plus the use of Terphenazine. The results indicated that children who were diagnosed as
having neurotic symptoms were far more responsive to the psychotherapy treatment than were the hyperkinetic children. Only about 15
percent of the hyperactive/hyperkinetic children reportedly improved
under the psychotherapy treatment. No evidence was found for any
improvement under conditions of psychotherapy and placebo treatment or psychotherapy and the active drug treatment.

Eisenberg, L., Lachman, R., Molling, P.A., Lockner, A., Mizelle,
J.D., and Conners, C.K.: A psychopharmacologic experiment in
a training school for delinquent boys: Methods, problems and
findings. *Am J Orthopsychiatry, 33*:431-447, 1963.

Delinquent Negro males were subjected to several experimental conditions—dextroamphetamine drug therapy, placebo drug therapy and observation with no drug treatment. Although there was a significant placebo effect, the houseparents and classroom teachers reported the greatest level of improvement under the central nervous system stimulant drug treatment.

Ellis, M.H., Witt, T.A., Reynolds, R., and Sprague, R.L.: Methylphenidate and the activity of hyperactives in the informal setting. *Child Devel, 45:*217-220, 1974.

Nine children, ages eight to ten years, in whom a trial period of methylphenidate therapy had been judged beneficial, were evaluated under varying dosages of methylphenidate. The purpose of this study was to determine whether the drug was capable of altering the activity of hyperactive children in a play situation. Data were obtained under double-blind controlled conditions through the use of a camera system. The conclusions drawn were that methylphenidate has little effect on the behavior of hyperactive children in nonstructured situations. It was suggested that the environment plays a strong role in determining whether or not the drug will be effective.

Epstein, L.C., Lasagna, L., Conners, C.K., and Rodriguez, A.: Correlation of dextraoamphetamine excretion and drug response in hyperkinetic children. *J Nerv Ment Dis, 146:*136-146, 1968.

In an effort to tap the interaction between the responses of children under dextroamphetamine and the clinical etiology of hyperkinesis, a sample of hyperactive children was evaluated under the central nervous system stimulant drug. Although all of the hyperactive subjects displayed improvement in the areas of fine motor coordination, Porteus-Maze test functioning and verbal abilities, the organic population displayed the most significant improvement.

Fish, B.: Drug Therapy and child psychiatry: Pharmacological aspects. *Compr Psychiatry, 1:*212-227, 1960.

Fish reported that amphetamine therapy is effective with only a small percentage of those children referred to clinics because of behavioral disorders. Central nervous system stimulant drug treatment was found to be most effective in children with overt behavioral disorders, and then most effective in that group of subjects who were the most mature and organized. In addition, the most dramatic responses were reported in children with school phobia and sexual preoccupations.

Fish, B.: The "one child, one drug" myth of stimulants in hyperkinesis. *Arch Psychiatry, 25*:193-203, 1971.

An admonition is delivered indicating that there is no one hyperactive child and, thus, no one specific intervention strategy that is best. Although the use of stimulant drugs may be effective with some children, they are not an efficient approach with others. It was also noted that the lack of a precise definition of the hyperactive/hyperkinetic syndrome adds to the difficulty of making an adequate diagnosis, and thus prescribing appropriate intervention techniques. The confusion surrounding the etiology of hyperactivity, especially minimal brain dysfunction, was also discussed.

Freeman, R.D.: Drug effects on learning in children: A selective review of the past thirty years. *J Spec Educ, 1*:17-44, 1966.

A review of drug research with children was aimed at identifying some of the methodological problems that are inherent in this type of research. Specifically, these problems and experimental issues were related to classroom and learning situations. In addition to a methodological review, an extensive drug research review was also given.

Geller, S.J.: Comparison of a tranquilizer and psychic energizer. *JAMA, 174*(5):481-484, 1960.

Geller was responsible for one of the first controlled, double-blind studies that attempted to evaluate the use of drug therapy with hyperactive children. A comparison made between a tranquilizing drug, a central nervous system stimulant drug and a placebo drug indicated that the three treatments brought about significant changes. The tranquilizing drug was found to be the most effective medication in reducing tension while the stimulant medication was found to be the most educationally useful.

Glick, B.S., and Margolis, R.: A study of the influence of experimental design on clinical outcome in drug research. *Am J Psychiatry, 118:*1087-1096, 1962.

A study of the influence of experimental design on clinical outcome in thirty-four published research reports indicated that those studies which included within their design a double-blind placebo, controlled technique had a significantly lower clinical improvement rate than did those which did not. It was also reported that long-term studies resulted in a significantly higher clinical improvement rate than did short-term studies, suggesting that both duration and degree of control are meaningful variables in determining clinical outcome.

Grant, G.R.: Psychopharmacology in childhood emotional and mental disorders. *J Pediatr,61:*626-637, 1962.

In a methodological criticism of much of the drug research conducted, it was suggested that criteria need to be established to validate the fact that drug therapy does in fact have a direct influence on the behavior of problem children. It was suggested that there needs to be an accurate, consistent, reliable and effective measure of the behavior that is under focus; populations which are large enough to allow for inferential parametric statistical procedures to be used; random assignment of subjects to various conditions; and the removal of basic resources of internal invalidity.

Knights, R.M., and Hinton, G.G.: The effects of methylphenidate (Ritalin) on the motor skills and behavior of children with learning problems. *J Nerv Ment Dis, 148*(6):643-653, 1969.

Children receiving methylphenidate treatment were reported to display a significantly greater degree of improvement than a placebo group on both motor skill test results and behavioral rating scales. Inferences drawn from this finding were that the results were attributable to an increased attention span rather than increased motor speed or control. In addition, the subjective behavioral scales completed by parents and teachers, which indicated an increased ability to attend, were interpreted to indicate improved motor control secondary to a greater ability to pay attention. Although it was reported that there was a significant placebo effect, both the parents and the teachers rated the active drug group as being less distractible and more attentive.

Knobel, M.: Diagnosis and treatment of psychiatric problems in children. *J Neuropsychiatry, 1:*82-91, 1959.

An uncontrolled study supported the therapeutic role of central nervous system stimulant drugs in treating and educating behavior problem children. Sixty-five percent of the behavior problem children sample in the study displayed definite improvement in behavior while under the influence of drugs. It was suggested that these drugs bring about a symptomatic improvement in behavior which sets off a chain reaction of modified attitudes such as better acceptance, understanding and tolerance by teachers and changes in peer relationships.

Knobel, M.: Psychopharmacology for the hyperkinetic child. *Arch Gen Psychiatry, 6:*198-202, 1962.

Knobel suggested that family or parental attitudes toward drug treatment may dictate the success or failure of a drug intervention program or even vary the results of such a program. Specifically, he concluded that a child or parent's "anti-drug effect" can significantly modify the final results of a drug strategy approach for dealing with the hyperactive child.

Knobel, M., Mohamed, S., and Pasqualini, G.: Pharmacological treatment of behavior disorders in children. *Int J Neuropsychiatry, 2:*660-666, 1966.

A replication of earlier suggestions that environmental influences are strong variables that can influence the pharmacological treatment of children was presented by Knobel et al. It was reported that negative expectations can produce negative side effects and reactions while favorable attitudes (placebo attitudes) can improve the favorable influence of a particular drug. It was reported that children of mothers harboring antidrug attitudes many times manifested toxic side effects, even in those cases where the children were receiving a placebo drug.

Kugel, R.B., and Alexander, T.: The effect of a central nervous system stimulant (Deanol) on behavior. *Pediatrics, 40*:651-655, 1963.

Kugel and Alexander reported that a group of hyperactive children were found to show nonsignificant differences under the influence of deanol and placebo drugs. Interviews indicated that over 50 percent of the children included in this study were reported to be significantly improved while on the placebo drugs.

Lasagna, L., Lateis, V., and Dohan, J.L.: Further studies on the pharmacology of placebo administration. *J Clin Invest, 37*:533-537, 1958.

Subjective responses of children under placebo treatment were found to be similar to characteristics found in the use of active drugs. Reports of "peak effects," "cumulative effects" and "carry-over effects" were all reported under placebo administration.

LaVeck, G.D., and Buckley, P.: The use of psychopharmacologic agents in retarded children with behavior disorders. *J Chron Dis, 13*:174-183, 1961.

LaVeck and Buckley reported nonsignificant differences in the behavior responses of exceptional children as a function of deanol, a central nervous system stimulant, and a placebo drug. Although the study was conducted with a retarded population, the investigators inferred that this pattern may also hold for a nonretarded population.

Lytton, G.J., and Knobel, M.: Diagnosis and treatment of behavior disorders in children. *Dis Nerv System, 20*(8):334-340, 1959.

Lytton and Knobel suggested that methylphenidate (Ritalin) has an influence on the cerebral cortex and that it can produce a "maturing effect" which can result in increased efficiency in overall cognitive functioning. It was suggested that the behavioral disorders encountered by school officials and parents basically have an organic etiology which can successfully be remediated through the use of central nervous system stimulant drugs.

McConnell, T.R., Cromwell, R.L., Bailer, I., and Son, C.D.: Studies in activity level: Effects of amphetamine drug administration on the activity level of retarded children. *Am J Ment Defic, 68*:647-651, 1964.

In a controlled, triple-blind study with retarded children, it was reported that there were no significant activity level changes as measured by a ballistograph and child rating scales under conditions of amphetamine administration. It was also reported that several subjects who were removed from the study because the drug was ostensibly thought to be precipitating excessively active ward behavior were on a placebo dosage at the time of the reported overactivity.

Millichap, J.G., Aymet, F., Sturgis, L.H., Larsen, K.W., and Egan, R.A.: Hyperkinetic behavior and learning disorders. *Am J Dis Child, 16*(3):235-244, 1968.

Methylphenidate treatment was reported to have a positive effect on the perceptual performance of hyperactive and learning disabled children. Significantly decreased actometer readings were also reported under drug treatment. A significant placebo effect equal to that of the active drug was also reported under certain conditions.

Millichap, J.G., and Boldrey, E.E.: Studies in hyperkinetic behavior. *Neurology, 17*(5):467-471, 1967.

Methylphenidate, phenobarbital and placebos were employed to evaluate the influence of drugs on the activity levels of children. Data indicated a significant difference between the methylphenidate and the placebo treatment, with activity being significantly reduced under the active medication.

Robin, S.S., and Bosco, J.J.: Ritalin for school children: The teacher's perspective. *J School Health, 63*:624-628, 1973.

Robin and Bosco's study focused on an examination of the attitudes and beliefs about the central nervous system stimulant drug Ritalin and the function of the educator in defining his role in working with children who are candidates for taking the drugs or who are already being administered the medication. One hundred and fifty elementary school teachers were administered a questionnaire regarding the drug Ritalin. Interestingly enough, most of the teachers were aware of the drug and its intended purpose. In addition, most of the attitudes of the teachers toward the use of the drug Ritalin were favorable. Few teachers voiced strong opposition to the use of the drug. Since the drug Ritalin is so closely connected with the classroom performance of the hyperactive child, the article focussed closely on the implications that it has for teachers and other educators.

Safer, D.J., and Allen, R.P.: Factors influencing the suppressant effects of two stimulant drugs on the growth of hyperactive children. *Pediatrics, 51*:660-667, 1973.

Safer and Allen designed a study to evaluate the effects of central nervous system stimulant drugs on the height and weight of hyperactive children; it revealed significant differences for the children on drugs when compared with those who were not on the medication. The hyperactive children who had been on central nervous system stimulant drugs for two or more years were compared with hyperactive children who had been advised to take drugs but who had not done so because of parental objections. Specific data indicated that the children on dextroamphetamine drugs lost an average of twenty percentile points in weight and thirteen percentile points in height. Those hyperactive students taking multiple dosages of methylphenidate were also found to lose in the area of height and weight. It was concluded that there were significant differences in the various central nervous system stimulant drugs that are administered hyperactive children and their dosages on the growth rate.

Satterfield, J.H., Cantwell, D.T., Saul, R.E., Lesser, L.I., and Pedosin, R.L.: Response to stimulant drug treatment in hyperactive children: Prediction from EEG and neurological findings. *J Autism and Child Schizo, 3*:36-48, 1973.

In an attempt to correlate the responsiveness to treatment with methylphenidate in a group of fifty-seven hyperactive children with EEG and neurological findings, teacher ratings were obtained before and after a three-week drug treatment period. The results indicated that 68 percent of the subjects had greater than 30 percent improvement on the posttreatment teacher rating scale. Eight subjects improved less than 30 percent and ten subjects declined on the teacher rating scale while under the drug treatment. Some of the conclusions drawn were that those children diagnosed as hyperactive who have abnormal neurological and EEG findings have a greater likelihood of responding positively to central nervous system stimulant drug treatment.

Schnackenberg, R.C.: Caffeine as a substitute for schedule II stimulants in hyperkinetic children. *Am J Psychiatry, 13:*796-798, 1973.

In a study on the effects of substituting caffeine for central nervous system stimulant drugs with hyperactive children, eleven subjects who had developed annoying side effects to methylphenidate were placed on the alternative drug. This alternative was delivered in the form of two cups of coffee a day following a three-week drug-free period. The effects of his change were measured by administering a rating scale to the classroom teachers of the subjects. Results indicated that the effects of caffeine were virtually the same as those of the active drug methylphenidate. It was concluded that because of the lower cost and reduced number of side effects, caffeine may be a therapeutic substitute for active central nervous system stimulant drugs.

Sprague, R.L., Barnes, K.R., and Werry, J.S.: Methylphenidate and thioridazine: Learning, reaction time, activity and classroom behavior in disturbed children. *Am J Orthopsychiatry, 40*(4):615-628, 1970.

Methylphenidate was reported to bring about a significant increase in the ability to respond correctly and a decrease in the hyperactivity of disturbed children. Teachers and other professional staff also subjectively supported the positive influence of the drug by noting that the children were more cooperative in and out of the classroom while under the drug treatment.

Sulzbacher, S.I.: Psychotropic medication with children: An evaluation of procedural biases in results of reported studies. *Pediatrics, 51:*513-517, 1973.

A review was given of 753 studies published between 1937 and 1971 on the effects of drug intervention techniques on learning and behavior in children. Each study was evaluated on the research design employed, the measures of change that were used, and whether the clinical results were statistically significant. Results indicated that the research design employed and the measures utilized exerted a strong biasing influence on the degree of reported significance in the various intervention strategies. It was concluded that an individual analysis is necessary to determine if the use of drugs is the most efficient intervention strategy for a given child and that clinically-relevant behaviors are employed as dependent measures in judging the effectiveness of the medications.

Sykes, D.H., Douglas, V.I., Gabrielle, W., and Minde, K.K.: Attention in hyperactive children and the effect of methylphenidate (Ritalin). *J Child Psychol Psychiatry, 12:*129-139, 1971.

Hyperactive children under methylphenidate treatment were reported to be able to detect more significant stimuli and to make fewer errors or impulsive responses than were a similar group of subjects receiving placebo treatment. It was inferred that this phenomenon was a function of the drug's ability to provide the children with skill in more effectively evaluating stimuli and inhibiting responses.

Weiss, G., Werry, J., Minde, K., Douglas, V., and Sykes, D.: The effects of dextroamphetamine and chlorpromazine on behavior and intellectual functioning. *J Child Psychol Psychiatry, 9:*145-156, 1968.

A double-blind uncrossed study confirmed earlier findings that dextroamphetamine treatment can improve the behavior of hyperactive children. In addition, the comparison study indicated that chlorpromazine had a moderately beneficial influence on the majority of the hyperactive children while dextroamphetamine had a more variable effect, with several children displaying no improvement at all. However, of the children benefiting from the dextroamphetamine (approximately 60%), the improvement was felt to be superior to that of chlorpromazine.

Werry, J.S., Weiss, G., Douglas, V., and Martin, J.: Studies on the hyperactive child. III: The effect of chlorpromazine upon behavior and learning ability. *J Am Acad Child Psychiatry, 5:*292-312, 1966.

A double-blind study using thirty-nine hyperactive children of normal intelligence demonstrated that a tranquilizing drug (chlorpromazine) was significantly superior to a placebo in reducing the level of activity in the children. It was noted that other behavioral symptoms were not as amenable to the drug treatment as were the direct bodily movements of the children. Even though the active drug was significantly superior to the placebo, there was a significant placebo effect. In over half the placebo group there was a definite improvement in behavior.

Winsberg, D.G., Dialer, I., Kupietz, S., and Tobias, J.: The effects of imipramine and dextroamphetamine on behavior of neuropsychiatrically imparied children. *Am J Psychiatry, 128:*1425-1431, 1972.

In an investigation of whether the drug imipramine could be effectively substituted as a stimulant drug free of noxious side effects, forty-one aggressive and hyperactive children were treated with the drugs, imipramine, placebo and dextroamphetamine. Results indicated that the degree of hyperactivity decreased in the subjects under both the active drug ingredients, and that the degree of inattention was significantly reduced as a function of the drug imipramine. In addition, it was noted that the toxic side effects frequently accompanying central nervous system stimulant drugs were significantly reduced with imipramine.

Wolf, F., and Pinsky, R.H.: Effects of placebo administration and occurrence of toxic reactions. *JAMA, 155*(4):339-341, 1954.

Approximately the same degree of improvement was noted in a group of hyperactive, behaviorally disordered subjects under the influence of placebo and central nervous system stimulant medication. This study emphasized the physiological effects of the placebo treatment.

Zimmerman, F.T., and Burgemeisten, B.B.: Action of methylphenidate (Ritalin) and reserpine in behavior disorders in children and adults. *Am J Psychiatry, 155*:323-328, 1968.

Matched groups of children were administered an intelligence test, followed by six months of drug therapy. Although no significant improvement in intelligence was noted, approximately 66 percent of the children were reported to have made behavioral improvements.

Zrull, J.P., Westman, J.C., Arthur, B., and Rice, D.L.: A comparison of Diazepam, D-amphetamine and placebo in the treatment of hyperkinetic syndrome in children. *Am J Psychiatry, 121:* 388-389, 1964.

It was reported that D-amphetamine was a treatment strategy that tended to be more effective than either a placebo treatment or Diazepam drug treatment in relieving manifestations of hyperactivity. Interestingly enough, the placebo drug was more effective than the diazepam.

Behavioral Techniques for Dealing with the Hyperactive Child

Allen, E.J., and Henkel, L.B., Harris, F.R., Baer, D.M., and Reynolds, N.J.: Control of hyperactivity by social reinforcement of attending behavior. *J Educ Psychol, 58*:231-237, 1967.

An investigation of whether or not adult attention could alter the pattern of hyperactivity in a four-year-old child was conducted. The procedures consisted of applying adult social reinforcement on those occasions when the subject maintained contact with a specific activity for a certain amount of time. Conclusions drawn from the data were that the making of adult attention contingent upon the child's maintaining his interest in a given activity were supported. This study is somewhat novel due to its successful use of nontangible reinforcers with a preschool child.

Becker, W.C., Madsen, C.H., Arnold, C.R., and Thomas, D.R.: The contingent use of teacher attention and praise in reducing classroom behavior problems. *J Spec Educa, 1:287-307, 1967.*

Ten "problem children" identified through a teacher referral system and, later, direct observation were placed under systematic behavioral conditions consisting of teacher attention contingent upon the subject manifesting appropriate behaviors. The results of the investigation demonstrated that the various teachers selected for the program were effectively able to employ behavioral principles to modify the behavior of specific children. The use of differential social reinforcement was found to be effective in modifying not only the behavior associated with hyperactivity, but also other deviant classroom behaviors.

Doubros, S.G., and Daniels, G.J.: An experimental approach to the reduction of overactive behavior. *Beh Res Ther, 4:251-258,* 1966.

A description of six mentally retarded, hyperactive males who were observed in a playroom setting is provided. The subjects were observed in the playroom over a two-week period. These observational sessions were used to construct a checklist of hyperactive behaviors. Behaviors were chosen from among those which were most frequently emitted; these consisted of stationary body movements, locomotive behaviors, destructive behaviors and communication. During the experimental phase of the study, token reinforcers backed up by candy were given to the children for staying with one activity. The results indicated that not only were the experimental techniques effective in reducing hyperactivity, but also that the hyperactive responses were significantly above the baseline phase for the extension and follow-up phases of the study. An interesting sidelight in the study was the finding that the most hyperactive subjects were the subjects who were most amenable to treatment. Conclusions drawn from this particular study were that hyperactivity can be reduced and that play session can acquire a higher level of organization and meaningfulness for a child if structured appropriately.

Homme, L.E., DeBaca, P.C., Devine, J.V., Steinhorst, R., and Rickert, E. J.: Use of the Premack principle in controlling the behavior of nursery school children. *J Exp Anal Beh,* 6(4):544, 1963.

The hyperactive and other behavioral excesses of 3 three-year-old nursery school children were effectively brought under control by use of the Premack principle. Although it was noted that the application of the principle was done in a relatively unsystematic fashion, it was nonetheless found to be quite effective in controlling hyperactive and overactive behaviors in preschool children.

Kauffman, J.M., and Hallahan, D.P.: Control of rough, physical behavior using novel contingencies and directive teaching. *Percept Mot Skills, 36:*1225-1226, 1973.

Novel reinforcement contingencies and directive teaching were implemented with a six-year-old hyperactive and aggressive male who had poor language and speech development. Results indicated that when the teacher provided reinforcement for appropriate play activities, destructive and inappropriate behaviors were significantly reduced. When this reinforcement was discontinued such behaviors became more frequent. It was also noted that during the use of a Distar program, rough, physical behaviors fell to near zero.

Luszki, W.A.: Controlling the brain damaged hyperactive child. *J Learn Disabil, 1:*44-52, 1968.

Parents are offered practical and nonesoteric techniques for controlling their school-age hyperactive children. Thorndike's Law of Effect was offered as a basic behavioral tool for aiding parents in controlling their hyperactive child. Environmental conditions, time-out procedures, play activities and general teaching procedures were specified.

Patterson, G.R.: An application of conditioning techniques to the control of a hyperactive child. In Ullman, L.P., and Krasner, L. (Eds): *Case Studies in Behavior Modification*. New York, HR & W, 1965.

An operant approach for controlling the classroom behavior of a nine-year-old hyperactive male is offered. Primary and social reinforcers were delivered through the use of a teaching machine apparatus that rewarded the subject for appropriate academic behaviors. Since the apparatus was manually operated there was a social reinforcement component to the delivery of the reinforcers, and thus a confounding of the variable that was most significant in reducing the subject's level of hyperactivity.

Patterson, G.R., Jones, R., Whittier, J., and Wright, M.A.: A behavior modification technique for the hyperactive child. *Beh res Ther*, 2:217-226, 1965.

A description of a conditioning procedure for increasing attending behavior in a ten-year-old brain injured, hyperactive male is offered. Categories of nonattending classroom behavior were developed via a classroom observation technique. Following this technique an apparatus was constructed whereby the experimental subject was able to receive auditory simulation when one of the specified behaviors did not occur for a given period of time. This auditory stimulus had previously been paired with the delivery of pennies or candy, and at the end of each trial period the subject receiving however many pennies or candy that he had earned.

The experimental subject was found to demonstrate a significantly decreased rate of nonattending behavior in the classroom while the nonattending rate for the control subject did not change markedly. This reduction was maintained over a four-week period of extension.

Pihl, R.D.: Conditioning procedures with hyperactive children. *Neurology, 17:*421-423, 1967.

Pihl reported two cases in which hyperactivity was successfully treated with operant conditioning techniques. The first case, a fourteen-year-old hyperactive male, was successfully conditioned to remain in his seat with the use of a token reinforcement system. In this case the subject was successfully able to achieve the goal of remaining in his chair for at least forty-five minutes under reasonable frustrating conditions with his therapist and mother. In the second case, a seven-year-old hyperactive male diagnosed as having signs of brain damage was successfully conditioned using a token reinforcement system in which points earned for staying in his seat could be exchanged for trading stamps. It was suggested that operant conditioning techniques can be successfully employed in dealing with hyperactivity in children and that once overactivity has been brought under stimulus control, other problems typically associated with hyperactivity can then be dealt with.

Twordosz, S., and Sajivaj, T.: Multiple effects of a procedure to increase sitting in a hyperactive, retarded boy. *J Appl Beh Anal, 5:*73-78, 1972.

In an effort to demonstrate that a nursery school teacher may be able to positively influence behaviors associated with hyperactivity, a four-year-old retarded male was placed on a token reinforcement behavior modification system. The data indicated that not only were desirable changes made in the area of enabling the child to maintain his placement in his seat for greater periods of time, but also that the development of other appropriate preschool skills and behaviors was brought about. It was concluded that this behavioral approach may be the avenue to appropriate functioning by reducing the behavioral phenomenon that most adversely affects the child's academic or pre-academic functioning.

Whitman, T.L., Caponigri, V., and Mercurio, J.: Reducing hyperactive behavior in a severely retarded child. *Ment Retard, 9*(3):17-19, 1971.

An operant conditioning procedure designed to reduce the hyperactive behavior in a six-year-old hyperactive female was presented. The results indicated that dispensing verbal and primary reinforcement was effective in reducing the out-of-seat behavior of this subject. This approach was quite successful even though it did not employ a punishment or time-out procedure along with the positive reinforcement.

Index

A

Academic achievement, 11, 12, 15, 55
Adapting materials, 148-51. *See also* Remedial methods
Additives, food, 35. *See also* Diet
Adolescents, hyperactive, 10, 12, 41
Alcoholism, 24, 59-60, 254
Allergies, 35-36, 52
Alternative models, 128-29, 154. *See also* Least Restrictive Environment
Amphetamines, 246. *See also* Drug therapy
Anxiety, 22-23
Assessment procedures, 8, 50-51, 61, 251-52, 257-63, 264. *See also* Measurement

B

Baseline observation, 56-61, 69, 84, 189
Behavior modification, 19, 33-35, 41, 61-62, 77-112, 117, 122, 136, 152, 154, 162, 179, 232
  material rewards, 86-87, 96-97, 111-12, 126, 133
Behavioral objectives, 29-30
Bender Gestalt Test, 207
Biofeedback techniques, 37-38, 42
Brain damage. *See* Neurological impairment

C

Chaining technique, 144
Child Rating Scale (CRS), 246, 258
Civil rights, 3. *See also* Drug therapy; Courts
Classroom management, 4-5, 27, 48. *See also* Educational management
Cognitive self-management, 42. *See also* Self-concept
Cognitive tempo, 20-21
  styles, 196-97, 199-203
Color, 111, 120, 150, 221-22
Conceptual Style Test (CST), 201-02
Conceptual tempo, 196-97, 199-203, 210
Conditional syndrome, 253-54
Contingency management, 134
Control group comparisons, 121, 162
Courts, 119. *See also* Civil rights
Curriculum for hyperactives, 30, 91, 121

D

Developmental syndrome, 254-55
Dexedrine, 69, 95. *See also* Drug therapy
Dextroamphetamine, 65. *See also* Drug therapy
Diagnostic process, 138-40, 141
Diet, 35, 42, 53. *See also* Additives, food
Drug therapy, 3, 14, 15-17, 19, 24-25, 30,

311

35, 39, 41, 47-73, 95, 116, 151, 160-61, 246
amphetamines, 246
Dexedrine, 69, 95
dextroamphetamine, 65
drug abuse, 32-33
guidelines, 32-33
research, 67-68
Ritalin, 32, 49, 65-66, 69
stimulants, 8-9
tranquilizers, 65, 102

E

Educational management, 115-55. *See also* Classroom management
Educational technology, 150-51
audio cassettes, 150
headsets, 132
tape recorders, 151
typewriters, 151
Ego states, 163-66. *See also* Transactional Analysis (TA)
Electroencephalograms, 16
Emotional disturbance, 3, 24, 95, 120, 122, 152, 167, 181-82
Encephalitis, 9, 15
Engineered classroom model, 122-29, 136
Environment, 15, 23-28, 30, 40, 41, 58, 72, 117-18, 120, 123, 152, 162, 166
family, 22
perceptual, 232
structured, 19, 118, 129-38, 151, 153
See also Scheduling; Reinforcement
Etiology, 160, 270

F

Family history, 51-52. *See also* Parents
Follow-up studies, 71-72
Feedback 21, 147, 151. *See also* Reinforcement; Punishment
Fernald Approach, 146

G

Games, 232
Genetic environment, 247, 254
Goal orientation, 232

H

Hyperactivity
behavioral characteristics of, 6-7
definition of, 6-8, 57-68, 115, 160, 244-45, 249, 250-51, 269
developmental, 19-22
measurements of, 8, 72, 141-42, 244-65
psychologically derived, 22-25
symptoms of, 3, 7-8, 19-21
syndrome of, 3, 7, 17, 244-45
Transactional Analysis and, 177-78, 183
Hyperkinetic. *See* Hyperactive

I

Impulse/reflectivity, 20-21. *See also* Reflection/Impulsivity
Incidence figures, 8-10, 269
Individualized instruction, 39, 120-21, 154, 233
Information processing, 14, 199-200, 218, 227, 229, 232-33
Instructional planning, 138, 154
Intellectual competence, 198
Intervention, 28-41
Inservice, 154
Irritability, 258
ITPA, 65

K

Kansas Reflection-Impulsivity Scale for Preschoolers (KRISP), 205-09, 214, 220-21, 230, 231

L

Labeling, 18, 48-49, 51, 161, 196, 249, 270
Learning Disabilities (LD), 3, 9, 173
Least Restrictive Environment, 119. *See also* Alternative models

M

Mainstreaming, 128, 154
Make a Picture Story (MAPS), 201
Matching Familiar Figures Test (MFF), 202-09, 212-15, 219-21, 225-29, 230, 231
Measurement, 8, 80-84, 244-65
behavioral, 72, 141-42